Dilfuzahon Mamarasulova

Cancer morbidity and organization of oncological care

Dilfuzahon Mamarasulova

Cancer morbidity and organization of oncological care

Monograph

ScienciaScripts

Imprint

Cover image: www.ingimage.com

This book is a translation from the original published under ISBN 978-620-8-00988-5.

Publisher:
Sciencia Scripts
is a trademark of
Dodo Books Indian Ocean Ltd. and OmniScriptum S.R.L publishing group

120 High Road, East Finchley, London, N2 9ED, United Kingdom
Str. Armeneasca 28/1, office 1, Chisinau MD-2012, Republic of Moldova, Europe
Printed at: see last page
ISBN: 978-620-8-19183-2

ANDIJAN STATE
MEDICAL SCHOOL

MAMARASULOVA DILFUZAKHON ZAKIRZHANOVNA

UDC 614.2:616-006

MONOGRAPHY.

ONCOLOGICAL MORBIDITY AND ORGANIZATION OF ONCOLOGICAL CARE

Andijan - 2024

TABLE OF CONTENTS

LIST OF ABBREVIATIONS

CI5	Рак на пяти континентах
БД	База данных
ВОЗ	Всемирная организация здравоохранения
ВОП	Врач общей практики
ДИ	Доверительный интервал
ЗН	Злокачественные новообразования
ЛПУ	Лечебно-профилактическое учреждение
МАИР	Международное агентство по изучению рака
МАРР	Международная ассоциация раковых регистров
МЗ	Министерство Здравоохранения
МКБ	Международная классификация болезней
ПКР	Популяционный канцер-регистр
РСНПМЦОиР	Республиканский специализированный научно практический медицинский центр онкологии и радиол
РУзб	Республика Узбекистан
p	Уровень значимости

INTRODUCTION

Currently, there is an increase in the incidence of malignant neoplasms (MN) all over the world, as well as in the Republic of Uzbekistan (RUzb). Thus, according to the data of the state statistical reporting in the Republic of Uzbekistan in 2021, 25,578 new cases of MN were detected. Over the last 5 years, the number of first-time detected cases has increased by 12.5%. The incidence of MN per 100,000 population in RUzb reached 74.0, which is 14.2% higher than 5 years ago. At the same time, breast, gastric and cervical diseases have taken the first places in the general structure of MN morbidity over the last few years.

According to the International Agency for Research on Cancer (IARC), malignant tumors are a common disease with a relatively high mortality rate worldwide. Projection data from IARC and the World Health Organization (WHO), available on the Cancer Today 2020 website, show significant differences in incidence rates by country. In countries in the European region, incidence rates range from 148.1 per 100,000 population (Albania) to 372.8 (Ireland) (standardized rates, Standard World). In Asian countries, rates range from 80.9 (Nepal) to 285.1 (Japan) per 100,000 population. The North American continent has higher incidence rates than the European region in both the United States (362.2) and Canada (348.0). According to IARC-WHO projections, Uzbekistan has an incidence rate of 108.1 per 100,000 population in 2020, which is higher than Tajikistan (89.7 per 100,000 population) but lower than Afghanistan (108.8), Pakistan (110.4), Turkmenistan (128.8), Kyrgyzstan (130.6) and Kazakhstan (166.9).

Currently in Uzbekistan there is a deficit of qualitative and reliable information on morbidity and mortality from diseases. State statistical forms provide prompt, but insufficiently specified and complete information on morbidity of the population of Uzbekistan. Form No. 7

"Information on diseases with malignant neoplasms" includes a limited list of localizations and only 5-year age breakdown. Form No. 35 "Information on patients with malignant neoplasms" also has a number of shortcomings, such as an even more limited list of localizations than in Form No. 7, lack of data on the sex and age of patients, and truncated data on special treatment. In both forms there is an inadequate accounting of tumor neoplasms in situ and primary-multiple MNs. In this connection, increasing the reliability of the information obtained from medical records requires urgent measures. One of the ways to solve this problem is to improve the level of organization of the oncological service through the introduction of population-based cancer registry.

The publication Cancer Incidence in Five Continents (CI5) is the main indicator for assessing the quality of cancer registries providing high quality and reliable information on newly diagnosed MN cases. Among the neighboring countries and CIS countries only 4 registries of the Russian Federation (Arkhangelsk, Karelia, Samara, Chelyabinsk), the Republic of Belarus and Ukraine provide information to this publication.

This research work for the most part serves to fulfill the tasks included in the Presidential Decree PP-2866 "On measures for further development of oncological care for the population of the Republic of Uzbekistan for 2017-2021 years" dated 04.04.2017 and PP-5130 dated 27.05.2021 "On further improvement of the system of providing hematological and oncological services to the population".

Correspondence of the research with the priority directions of development of science and technologies of the Republic.

This study was carried out in accordance with the priority directions of development of science and technology of the Republic of Uzbekistan - VI "Medicine and pharmacology".

Extent of study of the problem.

MN registration is one of the most important parts of the oncology service and the organization of cancer control in any country in the world. It is impossible to plan and further develop the cancer service without relying on reliable cancer registry data. A distinctive feature of the cancer registry is the availability of personalized data, i.e. detailed information about each patient with MN. Information from the cancer registry can be used in planning the financing of the oncology service: purchase of equipment, chemotherapeutic/targeted drugs, staffing, justification of the number of oncology beds in the branches of the center.

It is worth noting that there are two types of registers: hospital (hospital) and population registers.

Hospital registries store information about all patients with MN treated or diagnosed in a particular health care facility. A hospital cancer registry is mainly oriented towards administrative purposes and towards improving the quality of care provided to patients in a particular hospital.

Population-based cancer registries collect information on all new cases of MN occurring in a defined population in a geographic area. Data for a population-based cancer registry are collected systematically from several sources, including hospitals, death certificates, and laboratory services. Data from population-based cancer registries are the basis for estimating the prevalence of MNs and their trends over time. These data are critical for planning and evaluating cancer control programs in a defined population. This is their main purpose and determines their importance in cancer service organization and epidemiological and scientific research. The creation of a population-based cancer registry will not only help in organizing better and more targeted anti-cancer activities, but will also improve the quality and timeliness of the specialized treatment provided, to present their scientific research for publication in prestigious international journals, to participate in high-level international conferences and congresses, which will raise the prestige of the country in the world scientific arena.

It is worth noting that, according to WHO and IARC, there are currently more than 700 registries functioning in the world with different levels of population coverage, level of data quality and speed of development. The main studies on the quality of data collected by cancer registries are conducted by IARC (France), IARR (Japan), European Association of Cancer Registries - ENCR (Italy), Association of Cancer Registries of North European Countries - ANCR (Denmark), US National Cancer Institute (SEER) and others.

Relation of the thesis research with the plans of research works of the higher educational institution where the thesis was performed. This study was carried out on the basis of applied research grant of the Republican Specialized Scientific and Practical Medical Center of Oncology and Radiology of RUzb within the framework of the project FZ -202010191 (2022-2024) "Development of digital software product for complex assessment of oncoepidemiological state".

Purpose of the study

Development of methodology of population-based cancer registry in the Republic of Uzbekistan.

Research Objectives

Analysis of the organization of oncological care for patients with MN and the main statistical indicators in the Republic of Uzbekistan.

Creation of a population database of primary MN patients in order to identify errors and mistakes in case registration.

Formation of methodology, list of codifiers and reference books necessary for the work of the population stationer-register.

Determination of blocks of statistical indicators necessary to assess the state of oncological service and the quality of specialized medical care.

Object of the study. Methodology of registration of malignant neoplasms, list of variables mandatory for filling in registration forms.

Subject of the study. Accounting and reporting forms of medical documentation of primary patients with MN, international recommendations on registration and accounting of MN.

Research Methods. A retrospective method of research was used in the dissertation work. The main statistical indicators used in oncologic statistics were calculated according to the generally accepted methods. Processing of the obtained materials was carried out using Excel, IBM SPSS Statistics 23 programs. The database was created in the Access program.

Scientific novelty of the study

it has been proved that the detailed analysis of oncological service on the basis of calculation of rough intensive, standardized and age-specific indicators allows to optimize the work of oncological service at all stages of specialized medical care.

It was proved that identification of typical errors in staging of clinical stage, TNM and clinical group in registration of cancer patients on the basis of the created population base allows to evaluate the quality of registration of patients with malignant neoplasms and to develop programs to improve the quality of specialized medical care and treatment of cancer patients.

It was substantiated that for the first time formed methodological aspects of the population cancer registry, including 4 international reference books and 11 local codifiers necessary for adequate functioning of the population cancer registry, allow standardizing the coding and staging of oncological diseases to determine the correct tactics and individualization of treatment.

It was proved that the first developed complex of statistical indicators grouped by modules - indicators of primary morbidity of MN, indicators of mortality from MN, indicators of organization of dispensary registration, indicators of organization of treatment work, indicators of timely diagnostics, indicators of quality of preventive examinations of the population and screening programs, indicators of evaluation of distant results of treatment, allows to evaluate the state of oncological care, quality of services provided to the population, as well as to develop the following indicators

Practical results of the study

The assessment of the oncology service in the Republic of Uzbekistan has revealed shortcomings in the organization and planning of anti-cancer measures, the elimination of which makes it possible to improve the quality of medical services.

The analysis of the created population base allowed to reveal typical errors in registration of primary patients with MN at the territorial level, the elimination of which allows to improve the quality of treatment of patients.

For the population-based cancer registry system, 11 local-level codifiers have been developed and 4 international references (ICD-10, ICD-O-3, TNM, clinical stages) have been adapted.

A set of statistical indicators has been developed, the use of which makes it possible to improve the quality of epidemiological research, organization of oncological service and medical services provided to the population.

Reliability of the obtained results. The dissertation work was carried out in accordance with the requirements for medical and biological research, based on a sufficient amount of analyzed literature (including international requirements for the registration of MN cases and the creation of a population cancer-register), primary medical documentation with the use of modern methods of statistical processing of the results obtained.

Scientific and practical significance of the research results

The scientific significance of the results of the study lies in the creation of reliable data to improve the quality of scientific population and clinical research, as well as allow to optimize, individualize and improve the quality of treatment of patients with malignant neoplasms.

Practical significance of the dissertation work is to create a methodology for registration of MN cases according to international standards (IARC-WHO), which is necessary for functioning of the population cancert registry in the Republic of Uzbekistan.

Implementation of the research results

Based on the obtained scientific results to improve methodological aspects of population cancer registry in the Republic of Uzbekistan:

Methodological recommendations were approved: "Methodology for calculation of basic statistical indicators in oncology", developed based on the results of scientific research on the implementation of the methodology of population cancer registry in the Republic of Uzbekistan (certificate of the Ministry of Health of the Republic of Uzbekistan № 8 n-r/767 from 14.09.2021g). As a result, the quality of treatment provided to patients with malignant neoplasms has improved due to monitoring of early diagnosis and screening at the population level, early assessment of risk factors.

The results of scientific research to improve the methodology of population cancer registry in the Republic of Uzbekistan have been implemented in the practice of Samarkand and Fergana regional branches of RSNPMCRC (certificate of the Ministry of Health of the Republic of Uzbekistan № 8 n-z/320 from 06.10.2021g). Полученные результаты исследования внедрены в практику здравоохранения путем совершенствования методологии популяционного ракового регистра в Республике Узбекистан, формирования онкостатистических показателей, сгруппированных в 7 основных блоков, таких как показатели первичной заболеваемости злокачественными новообразованиями, показатели смертности от злокачественных новообразований, показатели организации диспансерного учета, показатели организации лечебной работы, показатели состояния своевременной диагностики, показатели качества пр

CHAPTER I . RELEVANCE OF CREATING A POPULATION-BASED CANCER REGISTRY (LITERATURE REVIEW)

The basis for the functioning of oncologic service and formation of anticancer activities in any country is the correct and complete registration of all malignant neoplasms (MN) [28, 54]. Based on the world experience in oncology, it should be noted that the correct registration of detected cases of MN is the basis on which the complex of measures to organize the fight against cancer is built [54]. None of the functioning and created anticancer measures will be effective without timely obtaining and analyzing qualitative and reliable data on the morbidity of MN population, assessment of the effectiveness of the applied treatment methods on the basis of studying their long-term results (analysis of cancer patients' survival rate), lethality, mortality and a number of other auxiliary indicators [1, 54].

§ 1.1 History of cancer registration

The oldest description of malignant tumors is found in the Egyptian papyrus of Edwin Smith, which describes breast cancer and states that there are no treatment methods for this disease (Fig. 1.1) [11, 16].

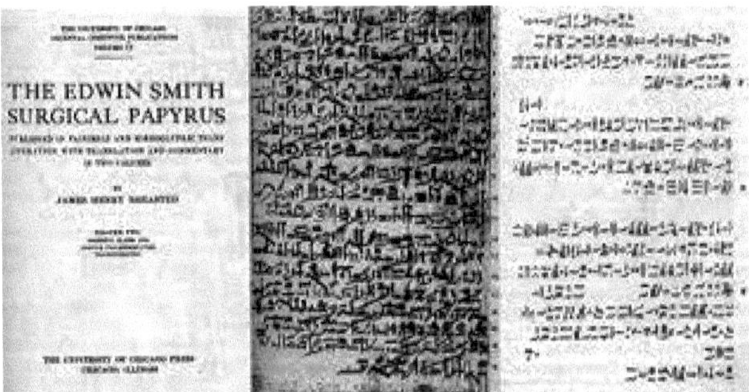

Fig.1.1 Edwin Smith's Egyptian papyrus

Hippocrates distinguished benign and malignant tumors, and also gave the first official name of the disease - crab, cancer (from Greek).

Many ancient physicians and philosophers not only described cases of the disease in their works, but also put forward theories of MN origin (lymphatic diseases, black fluid, trauma) [11].

Despite the fact that MNs have been known for a very long time, the science of oncology itself is a young science, which fully developed in the second half of the XX century. Clarification of the causes of the disease, development of new methods of treatment, diagnosis of MN at early and precancerous stages are the main tasks set before modern oncology. Fulfillment of these tasks is impossible without the organization of correct recording of cases and conducting scientific research on their basis in accordance with the principles of evidence-based medicine [8, 26].

The first attempt to register cancer diseases was made in London in 1728. The attempt was considered unsuccessful, as it was not possible to generate statistical data on MN incidence. In 1900 in Germany there was an attempt to register all cases of MN diseases. The method of registering MN was to send paper questionnaires to physicians around the country. A report on this questionnaire noted that only half of the completed questionnaires were returned. A similar method of registering MN was repeated from 1902 to 1908 in the Netherlands, Spain, Portugal, Hungary, Sweden, Denmark and Iceland. This method was also found to be unsuccessful [73].

Because of the unsatisfactory results of the above studies, Wood suggested in 1930 in the USA that mandatory registration of all MN cases was necessary. Later, a pilot project on mandatory registration of MN was started in Massachusetts. Due to incomplete coverage (about one third), this study was also considered unsuccessful [5, 58].

Continuous registration of patients with MN began in Mecklenburg in 1937 in order to obtain statistical information on cancer incidence. This was indeed the first step in collecting personalized information on patients with MN and for the first time made it possible to exclude repeated registrations and to determine the results of the study. The registration mechanism consisted in filling out registration cards (forms) and then sending these documents to the statistical office for verification and entering them into the file cabinet. This system of registration of MN worked quite well, as evidenced by the morbidity rate: from 1937 to 1938, about 200 new cases per 100,000 population [5, 58].

At about the same time, attempts were made in the United States to collect data on MN incidence [5, 58]. Information on MN incidence, mortality, and prevalence was collected in 10 metropolitan areas from 1937 to 1938. This national study was repeated from 1947 to 1948 and from 1969 to 1971. However, the fate of the patients included in these studies was unknown [5, 58, 104, 97].

The "oldest" cancer registry is the one in Hamburg. In 1926, a cancer registry was established with funding from a private medical organization. Already since 1929, this register has had an official status [50, 91, 92, 93, 94]. For the MN registration system, an active method was used, i.e.: several nurses collected information about new MN cases from health care facilities in Hamburg at a certain interval of time. This information was then sent to the central health department, where weekly reconciliation with death certificates took place [5, 58, 72, 104].

In 1935, a cancer research center was established in the United States (Connecticut), which began to register MN cases at the population level. The main purpose of this center was to conduct analysis of registered MN cases, including prevention, diagnosis, treatment, and mortality. The Connecticut Population Cancer Registry began statewide in 1941, retrospectively registering cases of MN since 1935. After that, other states in the United States and Canada established cancer registries in the early 1940s [5, 58, 104, 97].

In Denmark, a cancer registry was established in 1942 under the auspices of the Danish Cancer Society and is one of the first cancer registries at the population level. Information on MN diseases was collected passively. The task of the cancer registry was to collect information for follow-up of patients, to generate reliable statistical data on morbidity and mortality in order to evaluate the results of diagnosis and treatment; as well as epidemiologic studies [5, 58, 61, 104]. Since the mid-1940s, cancer registries have been launched in a number of countries, such as: England, Yugoslavia, Norway, Hungary, Finland, and Iceland [5,58].

In the USSR, the first attempts to register MNs and analyze information date back to the beginning of the XX century, after the All-Union Society for the Control of Oncological Diseases was established in 1908. The All-Union Society for Combating Oncologic Diseases was established in 1908. It is worth noting that only in 1953 in the USSR the system of registration of primary MN cases was finally formed and fixed by legislation. Also, the Ministry of Health of the USSR developed and approved accounting and reporting forms and basic principles of MN registration, which are still used in the post-Soviet countries [22, 24]. In the same years, in parallel with other republics of the USSR, the system of registration of MNs was developed in Uzbekistan.

Perhaps the most important impetus for the spread of the concept and foundations of the cancer registry was a conference held in Copenhagen in 1946, initiated by Dr. Klemmesen and the director of the Danish Cancer Registry (5, 58, 89, 96). It was recommended that cancer registries be established worldwide with the support of the World Health Organization (WHO). The basic principles of MN registration were also defined:

1. Information on cancer patients should be collected from as many countries as possible;

2. Data on cancer patients should be comparable with other countries;

3. Each country should have a central cancer registry to organize the collection of information;

4. There should be an international organization whose responsibility it is to monitor the collection of information and generate statistics from each country.

Four years later, WHO established a committee on MN registration and statistical processing, which developed recommendations for the establishment of cancer registries [97]. At the International Symposium Epidemiology and Demography of Cancer organized by the International Union Against Cancer in 1950, it was decided to establish a specialized center to study the burden of cancer. And already in 1965, the International Agency for Research on Cancer (IARC) was established as a specialized center for cancer research with the support of WHO. Subsequently, in 1966, the International Association of Cancer Registries (IARR) was established in Tokyo. IARR is a membership organization for cancer registries that collects and analyzes data on cancer incidence and also analyzes treatment outcomes of cancer patients [5, 22, 24, 58, 96].

The first report (Volume 1) of IARC and MARR "Cancer on Five Continents" was formed in 1966 and since then information has been compiled into a report every 5 years. Volume 12 is currently in preparation for publication[51]. Cancer on Five Continents is an invaluable source of information on the global prevalence of MN and Volume XI is more comprehensive than ever, providing high quality standardized data on cancers diagnosed between 2008 and 2012 [69].

Thus, the historical development of cancer registration can be clearly traced. Thanks to these activities, it is now possible to analyze cancer incidence, mortality, prevalence and survival rates in depth and compare them between countries worldwide [62, 69].

§ 1.2 Organization of oncology services in different countries of the world and in the Republic of Uzbekistan

Each country has its own health care system, which determines the conditions and procedure for providing highly qualified medical care.

For example, Australia used to have a network of organizations combined in the Cancer Network, but it did not fully cover the whole country, especially rural areas and remote areas. In order to improve access to medical care, it was planned to create a network of oncology facilities by retrofitting and reconstructing existing facilities. At present, the organization of oncological care in the country includes three levels, with a total of 24 specialized oncology centers:

Primary care, in the form of health care providers involved in screening

Cancer centers or hospitals at the regional level. Regional centers provide highly qualified treatment and diagnostics, as there is a direct connection with the main (capital city) centers.

Oncology clinics or university-based centers. They mainly provide expensive diagnostic and treatment methods, as well as research and training activities.

Since 1990, expert and consultative assistance to patients through telemedicine has been established, which has significantly improved the quality of medical services in remote regional cancer centers. Australia has also established a system of patient relocation/transfer thanks to subsidies from the government covering travel and accommodation costs [33, 87].

In turn, the National Cancer Institute (NCI) was established in the USA in 1937. Already in 1971, thanks to NCI, a national program to fight against cancer was created. NCI is engaged in organization and support of scientific research, evaluates new methods of MN treatment for their subsequent inclusion in practice, as well as provides support for the construction and reconstruction of oncological institutions. It is worth noting that in the USA almost all medical services are paid for, and most medical institutions are private [60].

The system of organization of medical care in Germany is the best among European countries. According to the law in Germany, the activity of all medical institutions, including oncology centers, is evaluated by quality control of medical services under the strict supervision of a special commission. On this basis, almost all medical institutions in Germany provide highly qualified care and are equipped with modern equipment [70].

Medical care in Canada, in turn, is subsidized by the state insurance fund. It is also possible to purchase additional services (private insurance) for dental care, nursing care and others. In Canada, almost as in Uzbekistan, a family doctor (GP) works in the primary care. The GP deals with the initial presentation of patients with MN. Then, for more in-depth diagnosis and treatment, the patient is referred to a regional oncology center. If highly qualified treatment is required, the patient is referred to the capital's (main) oncology clinic (100).

Poland has a system of compulsory health insurance, thanks to which the cancer care system is free of charge. The main cancer center in Poland is the Maria Skłodowska-Curie Institute of Oncology, which is under the control of the Ministry of Health. Moreover, practically all regions have oncology hospitals, inpatient clinics and departments, but not all of them are able to provide a full range of highly qualified medical care. It is worth noting that a significant number of medical services, including diagnosis and treatment, are provided in private medical institutions [56].

In turn, the organization of the oncology service in RUzb was based on the principles of Soviet health care, which provide for: unified, planned work of the oncology service; free, universally accessible, qualified care; preventive orientation (dispensary-type care).

It is worth noting that the oncological network of the Soviet Union was represented by 249 oncological dispensaries and more than 3500 oncological offices. The main link of the oncological network were dispensaries, organized in regional, oblast, republican centers, as well as in some large cities. Dispensaries were organizational and methodological centers in the territory of their service. Oncology offices at district/city polyclinics were also an important link of oncological care for the population.

In 1958, the first Research Institute of Oncology and Radiology was established in Tashkent on the initiative of Djura Majidovich Abdurasulov. In 2000, the Research Institute of Oncology and Radiology was transferred from the Academy of Sciences of Uzbekistan to the Ministry of Health (MOH) and renamed the Republican Cancer Research Center. In 2017, according to Presidential Decree No. 2866 of 04.04.2017, the center was renamed the Republican Specialized Scientific and Practical Medical Center of Oncology and Radiology (RSNPMCROiR), and regional oncology dispensaries and Tashkent City Oncology Dispensary were renamed as branches of RSNPMCROiR. An important document for oncology service is the Decree of the President № 5130 from 37.05.2021. RUzb "On further improvement of the system of providing hematologic and oncologic services to the population". This document serves as a basis for further development of the oncological service system in the country and improvement of specialized oncological care for the population [29, 30].

To date, the oncology service of the Republic of Uzbekistan represents a 4-level system, including:

1 - level - Ministry of Health of RUzb;

2 - level - RSNPMCo&R, which is an organizational and methodological center in oncology;

Level 3 - Regional oncology branches of RCHNPMCRC (13 branches), as well as Tashkent City Branch of RCHNPMCRC and RCHNPMCRC branch of the Republic of Karakalpakstan;

Level 4 - district oncologists in district/city medical associations (RMOs/GMOs).

Level 3 structural subdivisions are the main specialized therapeutic and preventive medical institutions involved in the organization and provision of oncological care to the population in a certain territory. The RSNPMCRC in its turn is the head oncological institution in the republic (Fig. 1.2) [29, 30, 34, 35].

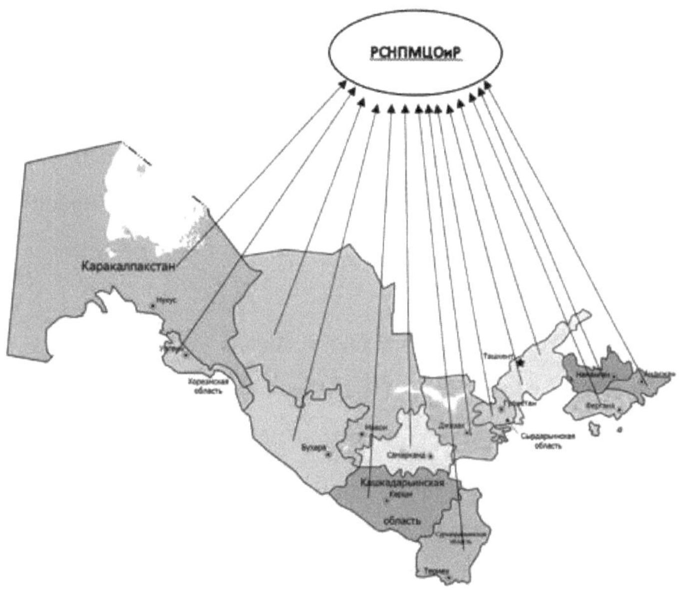

Fig.1.2 Oncological service of the Republic of Uzbekistan (levels 2 and 3)

An important link of oncological care to the population are oncology offices, which are created in the structure of district polyclinics. The doctor district oncologist should coordinate his work together with the oncology branch, provide methodological assistance in the organization of anti-cancer activities, including sanitary and educational work in the area of the oncology office.

When a patient visits a district oncologist, the doctor conducts an initial examination, refers the patient for the necessary examinations and, in case of suspicion of oncological pathology, refers the patient to the regional oncological branch of the RSNPMCRC, where an in-depth examination is carried out. If a cancerous disease is detected, a notification of a newly detected disease is filled out and sent within three days to the RMO/GMO at the patient's place of residence.

Specialized oncological care is provided at the branch in accordance with the "Standards of diagnostics and treatment of oncological patients" approved by the Ministry of Health of the Republic of Uzbekistan. For specialized high-tech treatment, which is not available in the branch of the RCHNPMCRC, the patient is given a warrant for treatment in the RCHNPMCRC [37].

After inpatient examination and treatment, the attending physician must fill out the following forms: an extract from the medical record of an inpatient with MN, if necessary, a protocol in case the patient is diagnosed with advanced MN, and a notice of first-time MN. All these documents are sent by mail to the RMO/GMO at the place of residence, where cancer patients are registered. Moreover, after treatment at the RSNPMCRC or its branch, the patient is referred to the district oncologist. In turn, the district oncologist registers the patient, provides counseling if necessary, fills out a control card of the cancer patient, which is kept for life and subsequently conducts dispensary follow-up [29, 30].

Properly organized work and accurate implementation of measures to improve cancer care for the population can reduce cancer mortality and neglect, improve survival and quality of life of cancer patients.

§ 1.3 Cancer situation in the world and in the Republic of Uzbekistan

In recent years, there has been an increase in the incidence of MN in most countries of the world, including the Republic of Uzbekistan. Thus, according to the state statistical reporting data, 21,976 new cases of MN were detected in RUzb in 2020. Over the last 10 years, the number of newly detected cases has increased by 15.6%. Breast, gastric and cervical cancers retain the leading positions in the overall structure of cancer morbidity [34, 35].

The WHO IARC projections available on the Cancer Today Global Cancer Observatory-IARC-2020 website show significant differences in incidence rates around the world. In countries in the European Region, incidence rates range from 148.1 per 100,000 population (Albania) to 372.8 (Ireland) (standardized rates, World). In Asian countries, incidence rates range from 80.9 (Nepal) to 285.1 (Japan) per 100,000 population. The North American continent has higher incidence rates (USA (362.2) and Canada (348.0)) than the European region. The projected incidence rate in Uzbekistan is 108.1 per 100,000 population, which is higher than in Tajikistan (89.7 per 100,000 population) but lower than in Afghanistan (108.8), Pakistan (110.4), Turkmenistan (128.8), Kyrgyzstan (130.6) and Kazakhstan (166.9).

The average mortality rate (standardized rate) in the world is projected to be 100.7 per 100,000 population in 2020. The lowest mortality rate was projected for Saudi Arabia (51.3 per 100,000 population) and the highest for Moldova (176.2). At the same time, in all countries the ratio of mortality to morbidity (based on standardized indicators) is quite high, which indicates the seriousness of the problem of radical treatment of MN. In the Republic of Uzbekistan, as in most Asian countries, this indicator exceeds 60% (Fig. 1.3) [51, 58, 69].

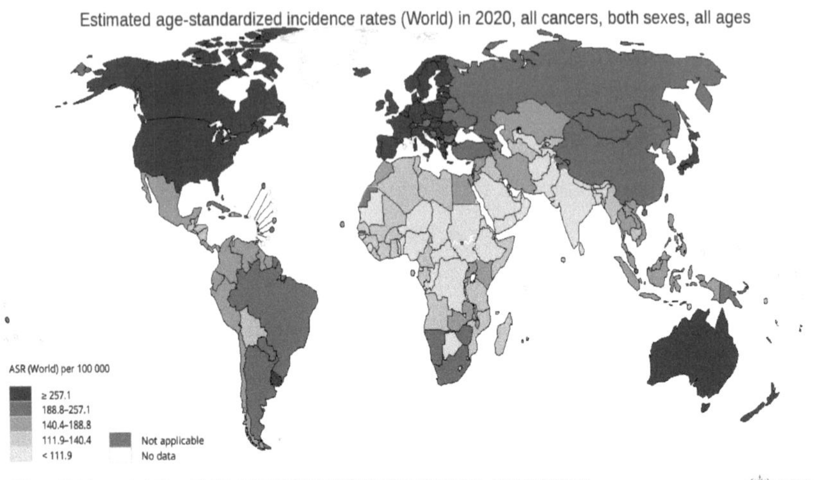
Estimated age-standardized incidence rates (World) in 2020, all cancers, both sexes, all ages
ASR (World) per 100 000
≥ 257.1
188.8–257.1
140.4–188.8
111.9–140.4
< 111.9
Not applicable
No data
All rights reserved. The designations employed and the presentation of the material in this publication do not imply the expression of any opinion whatsoever on the part of the World Health Organization / International Agency for Research on Cancer concerning the legal status of any country, territory, city or area or of its authorities, or concerning the delimitation of its frontiers or boundaries. Dotted and dashed lines on maps represent approximate borderlines for which there may not yet be full agreement.
Data source: GLOBOCAN 2020
Graph production: IARC
(http://gco.iarc.fr/today)
World Health Organization

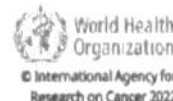
World Health Organization
© International Agency for Research on Cancer 2022

а

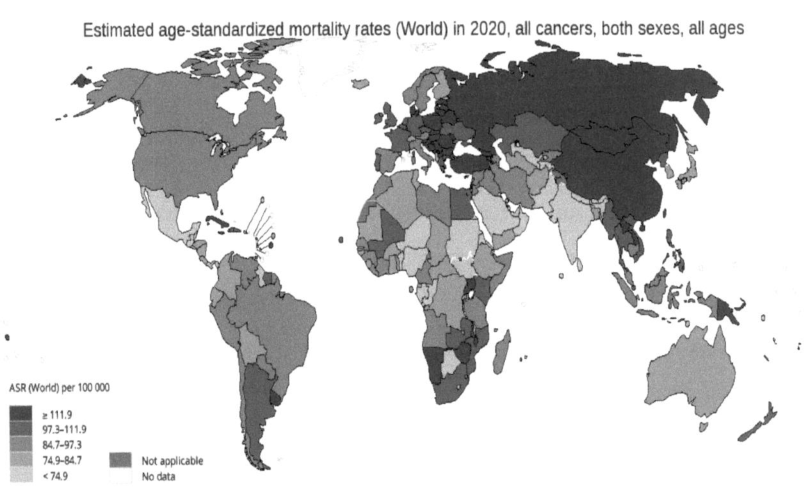
Estimated age-standardized mortality rates (World) in 2020, all cancers, both sexes, all ages
ASR (World) per 100 000
≥ 111.9
97.3–111.9
84.7–97.3
74.9–84.7
< 74.9
Not applicable
No data
All rights reserved. The designations employed and the presentation of the material in this publication do not imply the expression of any opinion whatsoever on the part of the World Health Organization / International Agency for Research on Cancer concerning the legal status of any country, territory, city or area or of its authorities, or concerning the delimitation of its frontiers or boundaries. Dotted and dashed lines on maps represent approximate borderlines for which there may not yet be full agreement.
Data source: GLOBOCAN 2020
Graph production: IARC
(http://gco.iarc.fr/today)
World Health Organization

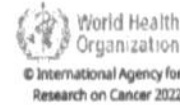
World Health Organization
© International Agency for Research on Cancer 2022

б

Fig.1.3 Incidence (a) and mortality (b) from malignant neoplasms (except skin melanoma) in selected countries of the world in 2020.

According to GLOBOCAN forecast data, at least 32,000 new cases of the disease should be detected in the Republic of Uzbekistan in 2020, while according to official statistics - 21,976, which indicates a significant under-recording of cases (Fig.1.4). Correct and comprehensive registration of all MN cases according to international requirements is possible only with the creation of a population-based cancer registry.

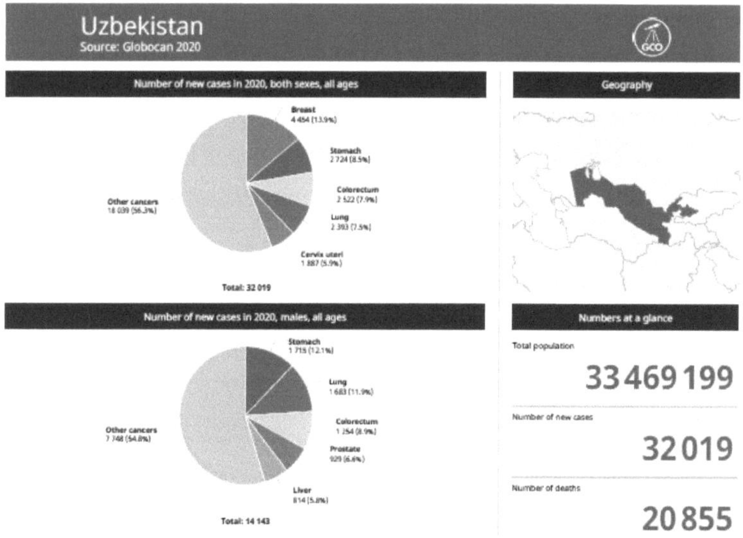

Fig.1.4 GLOBOCAN data for the Republic of Uzbekistan for 2020.

§ 1.4 Registration system for malignant neoplasms in different countries of the world

The capabilities, goals and objectives of hospital-based and population-based cancer registries need to be clearly distinguished. Hospital-based registries do not collect information on patients with MN tied to a specific area, but only register patients with MN diseases treated at a specific health care facility. Therefore, the purpose of hospital registries is to assess the performance, planning and management of a single health facility. Detailed information about patients in hospital registries, diagnostic and treatment outcomes are the basis for scientific analysis. However, hospital registries, as a rule, are not engaged in tracking the fate of patients and, due to the incompleteness of recording all cases of MN at the territorial level, are not able to provide information on MN morbidity, mortality from MN, dispensary and treatment results. For this purpose, population-based cancer registries are organized, which register all cases of MN diseases at the territorial level and make it possible to collect statistical data [24, 25, 54].

The main distinguishing feature of population-based cancer registries from statistical reporting is the availability of detailed information about each patient with MN. The availability of such information has two significant advantages: the possibility of adding and correcting data about patients in the process of their observation, which in turn improves the quality of the entered information; the possibility of long-term follow-up of patients' fate and the availability of survival data. Statistical reports, which are collected from primary medical records, have a sufficient number of deficiencies, due to the delay in obtaining information on registered cases and further refinement of it in the process of examination and treatment. The basic principle of oncologic statistics is to collect and correct data on patients with MN diseases within several years after registration. For this reason, almost all foreign articles publish not quite "fresh" statistical data [24, 54].

According to WHO and IARC, there are currently more than 700 registries in operation worldwide with varying levels of population coverage, data quality, and speed of development [51, 53]. All population-based cancer registries (PBRCs) can be assessed using five quality categories:

✓ high quality PCP (national) - covering more than 50% of the country's population;

✓ high quality PCR (regional) - coverage of less than 50% of the country's population;

✓ RCR (national and regional) - approaches RCR status and statistical indicators can be calculated;

✓ registration of MNs is underway - some registration of MNs is in place, but calculation of indicators is not possible;

✓ data on MN are not available or the situation with MN registration is unknown - data on the oncoepidemiologic situation in the country are not available.

As Figure 1.5 shows, there is no or unknown data on MN in Asian (including Uzbekistan) and African countries [51].

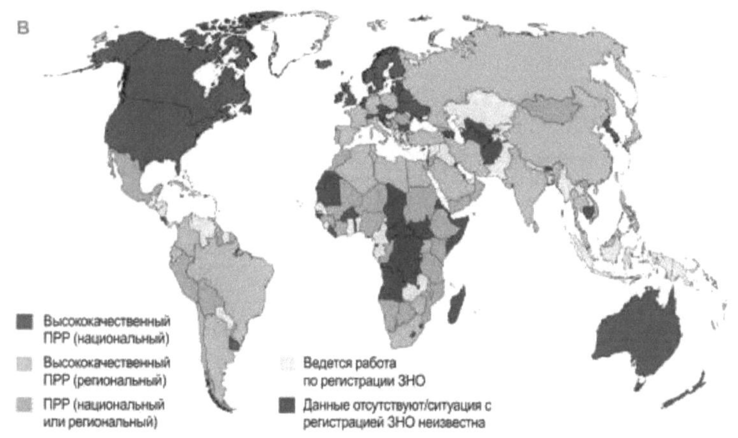

Fig.1.5 Existing worldwide chancery registries according to IARC data

Research based on general medical statistics alone is often quite limited, due to the inability to conduct cohort, case-control studies and to identify risk factors. Only general estimates suitable for hypothesis generation are possible. Population-based cancer registries provide the opportunity to conduct full in-depth scientific studies, with calculation of patient survival [24, 53, 54].

In turn, reliable and high-quality information on the incidence of MN worldwide is presented in CI5 every 5 years. The main purpose of this publication is to show comparable cancer incidence data for all countries around the world for which high-quality data from population-based cancer registries have been obtained.

For CI5 Volume XI, data from 483 cancer registries covering 636 populations in 90 countries were submitted. Data from 140 cancer registries representing 171 populations were excluded (Figure 1.6). The number of registries included for analysis varies from year to year. The number of registries (%) included in the CI5 Volume XI edition of the submission (by continent) are as follows: Africa, 23% (7/30); Central and South America, 69% (31/45); North America, 97% (69/71); Asia, 53% (97/182); Europe, 88% (127/143); and Oceania: 100% (12/12). The proportion of the total world population covered by Volume XI registries is 15%, with the following levels of coverage by continent: Africa, 1%; Central and South America, 8%; North America, 98%; Asia, 7%; Europe, 46%; and Oceania, 77% (51, 52, 55).

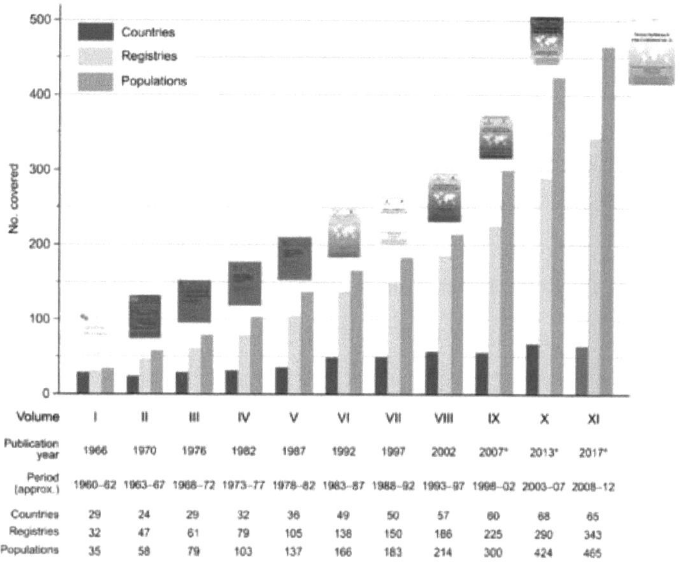

Figure 1.6 Data from Volume XI of CI5

All stationery registers included in the CI5 edition have been analyzed. More detailed analysis was performed for the following country registries: South Korea, Turkey, Kyrgyzstan, Austria, Belarus, Estonia, Latvia, Lithuania, Russian Federation, Ukraine. It is important to note that in South Korea and Turkey information on MN cases is collected by 8 registries (Fig.1.7). While in South Korea, information on MN cases is collected by 8 regional and 1 national registry, which receives information from both regional and hospital registries, in Turkey, information is provided by 8 high-quality regional registries [52, 86, 48, 101].

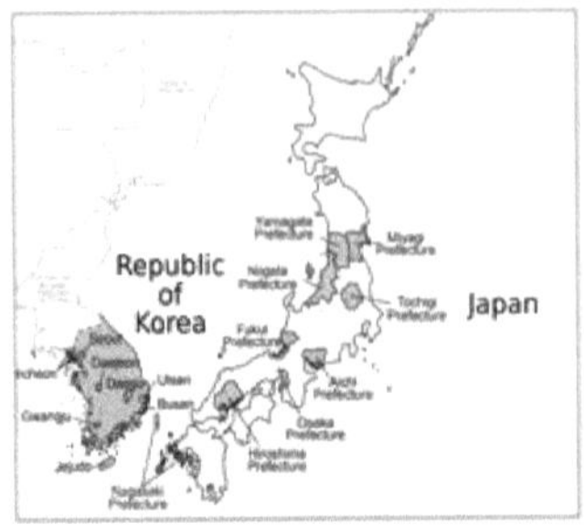

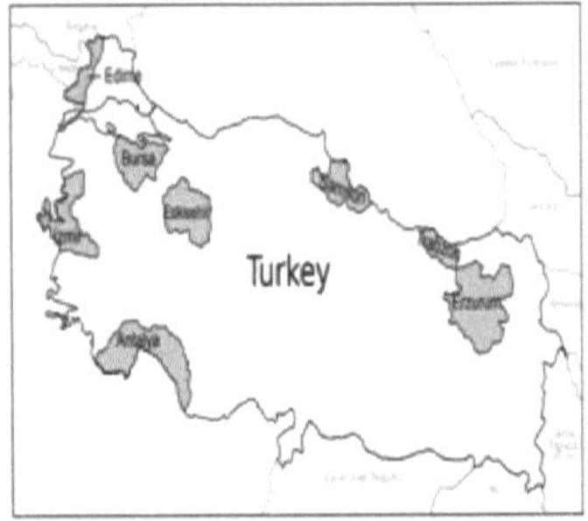

Fig. 1.7 Coverage of Kanzer registers in South Korea and Turkey (data from Volume XI of CI5)

Austria has 3 regional cancer registries and a National Cancer Registry, which collects information on all MN cases in the country from regional and hospital cancer registries (Figure 1.8).

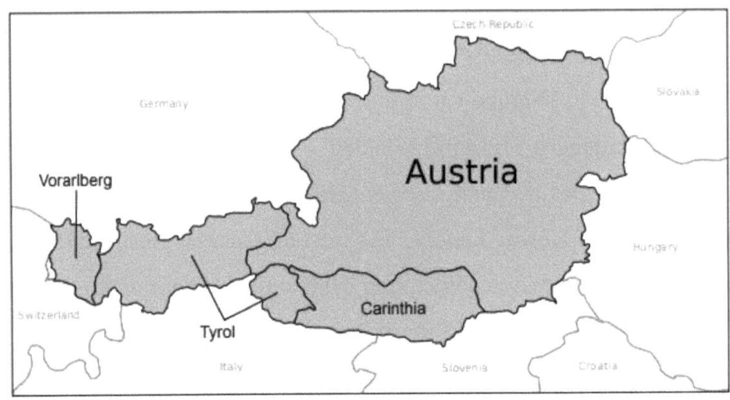

Figure 1.8 Coverage of Kanzer Registers in Austria (data from CI5 Volume XI)

Data on MN morbidity in the Russian Federation are obtained from 4 country registers (Fig. 1.9).

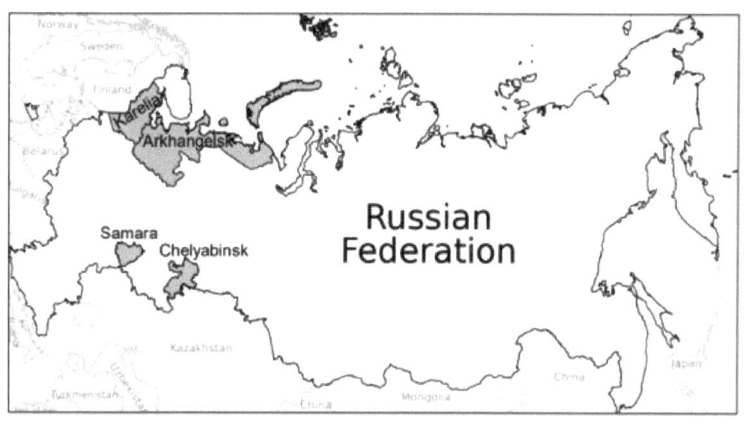

Fig.1.9 Coverage of Kancer Registers in the Russian Federation (data from Volume XI of CI5)

Table 1.1 presents information on the cancer registries included in the CI5 publication by year. The conclusion to be drawn from the information presented in Table 1.1 is that any cancer registry must provide high quality data for each CI5 publication. If a registry's data does not meet this criterion, the registry is not included in the publication. For example, data from a cancer registry in South Korea (Kangwa) were included in Volumes 7 and 8, but the registry was subsequently excluded from publication in CI5 Volumes 9-11. Also, the registries of St. Petersburg and Kyrgyzstan were accepted for publication only in certain volumes [82, 85, 95, 98].

Table 1.1.

Kanzer registers included in CI5 editions

Country	Region	Time period of CI5 editions						
		T1-T5	T6	T7	T8	T9	T10	T11
South Korea	Busan	-	-	-	1996-97	1998-02	2003-07	2008-12

	Daegu	-	-	-	1997-98	1998-02	2003-07	2008-12
	Daejeon	-	-	-	-	1998-02	2003-07	2008-12
	Gwangju	-	-	-	-	1998-02	2003-07	2008-12
	Incheon	-	-	-	-	1998-02	2003-07	2008-12
	Jeju	-	-	-	-	2000-02	2004-07	2008-12
	Kangwa	-	-	1986-92	1993-97	-	-	-
	Seoul	-	-	-	1993-97	1998-02	2003-07	2008-12
	Ulsan	-	-	-	-	1999-02	2003-07	2008-12
Turkey	Antalya	-	-	-	-	1998-02	2003-07	2008-12
	Bursa	-	-	-	-	-	-	2008-12
	Edirne	-	-	-	-	-	2004-07	2008-12
	Erzurum	-	-	-	-	-	-	2010-12
	Esquisehir	-	-	-	-	-	-	2008-12
	Izmir	-	-	-	-	1998-02	2003-07	2008-12
	Samsun	-	-	-	-	-	-	2008-12
	Trabzon	-	-	-	-	-	2005-07	2008-12
Austria	Carinthia	-	-	-	-	-	-	2008-12
	Tyrol	-	-	1998-92	1993-97	1998-02	2003-07	2008-12
	Voralberg	-	-	-	1993-97	1998-02	2003-07	2008-12
Belarus		-	1983-87	1988-92	1993-97	1998-02	2003-07	2008-12
Estonia		-	1983-87	1988-92	1993-97	1998-02	2003-07	2008-12
Latvia		-	1993-87	1988-92	1993-97	1998-02	2003-07	2010-12
Lithuania		-	-	-	1993-97	1998-02	2003-07	2008-12
RF	Arkhangelsk	-	-	-	-	-	-	2008-12
	Chelyabinsk	-	-	-	-	-	-	2008-12
	Karelia	-	-	-	-	-	-	2008-12
	St. Petersburg	-	1983-87	-	1994-97	1998-02	2003-07	-

	Samara	-	-	-	-	-	-	2008-12
Ukraine		-	-	-	-	-	2003-07	2008-12
Kyrgyzstan		-	1986-87	-	-	-	-	-

Of all the registers under consideration (Table 1.2), the oldest is the Estonian register, which started functioning in 1968; however, the data from this register were accepted for publication in CI5 (i.e., passed the quality and reliability checks) only in Volume VI (1983-1987). In 1973, the population cancer registry of Belarus began to function, and its data were accepted for publication in CI5 also in Volume VI. Thus, an average of 10-15 years passes from the moment of cancer registry creation to the moment data from it are accepted for publication, which once again confirms the complexity of developing a system of registration and registration of MNs according to international requirements [51, 96].

Table 1.2.

Summary of the stationery registers included in the CI5 edition

Country	Region	Information about the stationery registers included in CI5				
		Average annual population	Area	% population coverage	Start of operation of the registry (year)	Legislative/ administrative records
South Korea	National level	49 879 612	100 032	82	1980	yes
	Busan	3 536 355	764	95	1995	yes
	Daegu	2 488 813	775	82	1980	yes
	Daejeon	1 490 874	540	100	1998	yes
	Gwangju	1 438 340	501	95	1997	yes
	Incheon	2 728 573	1 029	98	1996	yes
	Jeju	565 812	1 848	-	2000	yes
	Seoul	10 151 175	605	100	1991	yes
	Ulsan	1 118 760	1 059	94	2001	yes
Turkey	Antalya	1 978 671	20 815	70	1995	yes
	Bursa	2 600 880	10 882	89	2000	yes
	Edirne	395 911	6 276	68	2004	yes
	Erzurum	776 042	49 324	64	2006	yes
	Esquisehir	766 549	13 925	89	2005	yes

	Izmir	3 916 765	11 973	91	1992	yes
	Samsun	1 247 979	9 352	65	2001	yes
	Trabzon	759 614	4 685	54	2003	yes
Austria	National level	8 367 787	83 879	-	1983	yes
	Carinthia	559 257	9 538	51	1987	yes
	Tyrol	707 670	12 648	-	1987	yes
	Voralberg	368 934	2 601	36	1978	yes
Belarus		9 492 600	207 600	100	1973	yes
Estonia		1 330 643	45 227	68	1968	yes
Latvia		2 063 852	64 589	100	1991	yes
Lithuania		3 094 863	65 300	67	1975	yes
RF	Arkhangelsk	1 235 854	766 513	75	1993	yes
	Chelyabinsk	3 482 299	88 500	82	2007	yes
	Karelia	655 929	180	79	1996	yes
	Samara	3 188 626	53 600	80	2003	yes
Ukraine		45 797 940	603 000	68	1989	yes

It should be noted that 100% population coverage of the register at the population level has been achieved in Latvia and Belarus, and at the regional level in Seoul and Daejeon (Republic of Korea).

Laws or regulations governing the registration of all MNs generally improve the quality of registry data by making information (or reporting) available to all facilities that diagnose or treat MNs, including those in the private sector.

All the registers considered in Table 1.3 differ in the number of variables required and sources of information. Thus, according to IARC-WHO international recommendations, the minimum set of data to be collected by a cancer registry is: patient data (personal identifier, full name, gender, date of birth, residential address) and tumor information (date of diagnosis, most reliable method of diagnosis, localization, morphological type, tumor behavior, source of information - outpatient card number, name of the doctor); basic set: more extended information about the patient, about the tumor (according to international requirements (ENCR) and classifiers (ICD-10 and ICD -O-3), information about the stage of the disease (TNM), primary treatment information (treatment started within 4 months after diagnosis), sources of information (all medical institutions involved in the treatment and diagnosis of MN), dispensary follow-up (date of the last patient follow-up, status (alive/dead), date of death). The basic data set can be expanded according to the capabilities and goals of the registry [49, 51, 53, 77, 102].

Table 1.3.

Information collection methods and international standards of the CI5 edition of the Chancery Registers

Country	Region	Information about the stationery registers included in CI5					
		ID	Ethnic group	Initial treatment	Observation	Observation method	International Standard
South Korea	National level	yes	no	Yes	yes	passive	IARC/IACR
	Busan	yes	no	Yes	yes	passive	IARC/IACR
	Daegu	yes	no	Yes	yes	passive	IARC/IACR
	Daejeon	yes	no	Yes	yes	passive	IARC/IACR
	Gwangju	yes	no	Yes	yes	passive	IARC/IACR
	Incheon	yes	no	Yes	yes	passive	IARC/IACR
	Jeju	yes	no	Yes	yes	passive	IARC/IACR
	Seoul	yes	no	Yes	yes	passive	IARC/IACR
	Ulsan	yes	no	Yes	yes	passive	IARC/IACR
Turkey	Antalya	yes	no	Yes	yes	active	IARC/IACR
	Bursa	yes	no	Yes	yes	active	SEER
	Edirne	yes	no	Yes	yes	active	IARC/IACR
	Erzurum	yes	no	Yes	yes	active	IARC/IACR
	Esquisehir	yes	no	Yes	yes	active	IARC/IACR
	Izmir	yes	no	Yes	yes	active	SEER
	Samsun	yes	no	Yes	yes	active	IARC/IACR
	Trabzon	yes	no	Yes	yes	active	IARC/IACR
Austria	National level	yes	no	Yes	yes	passive	ENCR
	Carinthia	no	no	Yes	yes	active	ENCR
	Tyrol	no	no	Yes	yes	passive	ENCR
	Voralberg	yes	no	No	yes	active	ENCR
Belarus	All of it	yes	yes	Yes	yes	active+passive	IARC/IACR
Estonia	All of it	yes	yes	Yes	yes	passive	ENCR
Latvia	All of it	yes	yes	Yes	yes	active	IARC/IACR
Lithuania	All of it	yes	no	No	yes	passive	IARC/IACR
RF	Arkhangelsk	no	no	Yes	yes	active+passive	IARC/IACR
	Chelyabinsk	yes	yes	No	yes	active+passive	IARC/IACR
	Karelia	no	no	Yes	yes	active+passive	IARC/IACR

	Samara	yes	yes	Yes	yes	active+passive	IARC/IACR
Ukraine	All of it	no	yes	Yes	yes	active+passive	IARC/IACR

The most important data sources for any Kancer registry are pathology laboratories, hospital records (both public and private hospitals), and death certificates. There is still a shortage of death certificates in low- and middle-income countries, mainly due to the poor quality of mortality statistics in general (South Korea, Latvia, Chelyabinsk).

Moreover, unique patient identification numbers are not used in Arkhangelsk, Karelia and Ukraine, ethnic group - Korea, Turkey, Austria, Lithuania, Arkhangelsk and Karelia, nature of primary treatment received - Lithuania and Chelyabinsk. Universal variables at the level of patient information as well as primary localization of MN and histology are not considered in the presented table, as they are almost always collected by Kancer registries and are mandatory for high-quality registries. Systematic observation of the vital status of registered patients is conducted in all registries under consideration. The difference is the method of observation - active or passive. Thus, in Korea, Austria, Estonia, and Lithuania, passive surveillance is used (health care workers fill out notification forms and send them to the registry), in Turkey and Latvia, active surveillance is used (cancer registry staff visit all medical clinics to obtain the necessary data), and in Belarus, Russia, and Ukraine, both active and passive surveillance are used [36, 45, 51, 53].

There are several international standards for registration of MN cases, such as SEER (Statistical Surveillance, Epidemiology and End Results Program) recommendations in Bursa and Izmir, ENCR (European Network of Cancer Registries) in Austria, Estonia, Arkhangelsk and Samara, and IARC/IACR (International Agency for Research on

Cancer/International Association of Cancer Registries) in the other registries reviewed [43, 46, 47, 51, 52, 103].

1.5 Characterization of the main statistical indicators in oncology

The system of oncologic statistics includes indicators that can be conditionally divided into two groups [7, 9, 24, 54]:

✓ Indicators used to estimate cancer prevalence (absolute numbers, extensive/intensive incidence and mortality rates).

✓ Indicators used to assess the effectiveness of anti-cancer measures (indicators). In many post-Soviet countries, in order to assess the performance of health care in administrative territories, the indicators of "outcome models" are used, the indicators of which are calculated according to generally accepted algorithms [4, 14, 21, 29, 30, 32, 34, 35]. These models allow us to give a generalized assessment of the state of oncological care in the regions, but do not allow us to detail the problematic aspects of work necessary for targeted planning of cancer control.

The main methods of assessing the quality of medical care and organization of the health care system in RUzb, as well as in other post-Soviet countries, remain: statistical analysis (indicators of state and departmental statistical reporting) and expert evaluation (expert examination of patients' medical records); sociological survey is used much less frequently (to determine patient satisfaction with treatment, quality of service, etc.). [29, 30, 34, 35, 40]. The statistical reporting forms submitted to the Ministry of Health of the RUzb contain insufficiently detailed information for the development and organization of anticancer measures. Most of the indicators reflect quantitative aspects of medical care rather than its quality. The need to supplement the existing indicators with indicators that will contribute to the solution of health care system tasks relevant for the nearest period becomes obvious [29, 30, 31, 34, 35, 39, 40, 41].

To address the issue of continuous improvement of the quality of medical care based on system analysis, many countries have developed national programs [78, 80, 81, 90]. To ensure the quality of medical care, decision-making based on in-depth analysis using appropriate quality assessment models of integral indicators and monitoring of the situation is important [40, 78, 79, 80, 90].

Integral indicators include the ratio of mortality to morbidity, mortality from MN, mortality, and survival rates. The analysis of these indicators allows comparative analysis and evaluation of the effectiveness of anticancer measures [3, 24, 25, 38, 42, 64].

There are commonly accepted indicators for evaluating various cancer control programs. Table 1.4 presents some programs and indicators for evaluating their effectiveness.

Table 1.4.

Indicators used to evaluate cancer control programs

program	Indicators
Primary prevention	Decrease in morbidity
Screening and early diagnosis	Reduced mortality
New diagnostic methods	Improving early diagnosis rates; Increased coverage of radicalized treatment; Decrease in one-year mortality; Reduced mortality
New therapies	Reduced mortality Reduced mortality Increased survival rate
Dispensary	Early diagnosis of recurrences Reduced mortality Increased survival rate

Summary

According to the world forecast data, at least 32,000 new cases of the disease should be detected in Uzbekistan in 2020, while according to official statistics - 21,976, which indicates a significant under-recording of cases. Correct and comprehensive registration of all MN cases according to international requirements is possible only if a population-based cancer registry is created.

The main distinguishing feature of population-based cancer registries from statistical reporting is the availability of detailed information about each patient with MN. The availability of such information has two significant advantages: the possibility of adding and correcting data about patients in the process of their observation, which in turn improves the quality of the entered information; the possibility of long-term follow-up of patients' fate and the availability of survival data. Statistical reports, which are collected from primary medical records, have a sufficient number of shortcomings due to the delay in obtaining information on registered cases and its further refinement in the process of examination and treatment.

Planning of anticancer interventions in RUzb, as well as analysis of cancer patient survival at the population level will become possible after the organization of a population-based cancer registry in the country according to international standards. In the framework of this study, work was carried out to develop a methodology for a population-based cancer registry in RUzb.

CHAPTER II MATERIALS AND METHODS

The development of the methodology of the population-based cancer registry was based on the IARC-WHO recommendations: sources of information on first-time cases of MN (accounting forms of the Ministry of Health of the Republic of Uzbekistan), coding and confirmation of cases (ICD-10 and ICD-O-3), diagnosis (laboratory and instrumental diagnostic methods available in the country), treatment methods (in accordance with national standards of treatment of MN patients), statistical indicators to assess the prevalence of MN and the quality of services provided to patients with MN.

§2.1 Analysis of the primary morbidity rate of malignant neoplasms

The material for studying the oncological situation in the Republic of Uzbekistan was the data obtained from the state reporting form on oncology (№7) "Information on diseases with malignant neoplasms" - the absolute number of first detected cases of MN in 2020.

To analyze the oncological situation for 2020 in Bukhara oblast, data from the state reporting form and personalized information from the primary documentation of the Bukhara branch of the RSNPMCRC were used. In addition to analysis of the total number of first-time cases, data on 1,584 primary patients were analyzed, including distribution by stage, TNM, calculation of crude, age and standardized indices. Standardization of morbidity rates was performed by direct method using the world population standard (World Standard).

§2.2 Structure of the population canzer-register

Based on the vertical system of organization of oncological service in the Republic of Uzbekistan, the structure of the Population Cancer Registry (PCR) is as follows (Fig. 2.1):

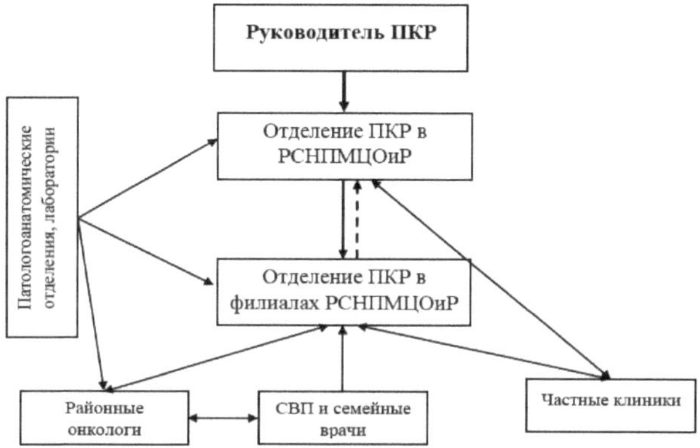

Fig.2.1 Structure of the population canzer-register

Head of the RPC - directly supervises all RPC units both in RSNPMCRC and in its branches, provides information on various issues related to both technical and oncological pathology: clinical oncology, epidemiology and statistics of oncological diseases at the request of the administration of RSNPMCRC, the Ministry of Health and other departmental organizations.

The RPC department in RSNPMCHC - controls the timeliness, quality and completeness of the information entered into the register database, provides advisory and methodological assistance to the staff of the RPC departments in the branches of RSNPMCHC, district oncologists, provides reporting information on the status of oncology service at the request of the head of the RPC, administration of RSNPMCHC, heads of regional branches, researchers, provides reporting information to the Ministry of Health.

PCR departments in the branches of the RSNPMCHC - exercises control at the regional level over the timely, qualitative and complete entry of information into the database of the register, entry into the PCR database of information on all first-time cases of MN and information on the methods of treatment and medical examination of patients assigned to the territory of the branch, provides consultative and methodological assistance to oncologists.

District oncologists - supervise the dispensary examination of oncological patients registered with MN, liaise with pathology departments, SVPs and family physicians, supervise the entry of first-time cases into the database.

SVPs and family physicians - if a patient is suspected of having a malignant neoplasm, refer the patient for follow-up examination to a district oncologist or to a branch of the RSNPMCHC and fill out a notification of a first-discovered MN.

Pathology departments - perform histological confirmation of the diagnosis, after which they send the results of the research to the relevant departments of RPCs and treating physicians. When a malignant neoplasm is detected after death (with or without autopsy), a notification of a first-detected MN is filled out.

Private clinics - fill out notifications of first-time MN cases and send to community affiliates or the district oncologist.

The organization of working groups in PCD departments should be based on the number of population in the assigned territory, taking into account the number of MN cases.

§2.3 Sources of information on cases of malignant neoplasms

Information on patients with MN in RUzb is collected and entered based on the following documentation:

- ✓ Medical card of an outpatient (form No. 025, approved by the order of the Ministry of Health dated 31.12.2020, No. 363);
- ✓ Medical record of an inpatient

✓ Extract from the medical record of an inpatient with malignant neoplasms (form No. 027-1/u, approved by the order of the Ministry of Health of 31.12.2020, No. 363);

✓ Notification of the first-time established case of malignant neoplasm (form No. 090/u, approved by the order of the Ministry of Health of 31.12.2020, No. 363);

✓ Protocol for the case of detection of a patient with a neglected form of malignant neoplasm (form No. 027-2/u, approved by the order of the Ministry of Health of 31.12.2020, No. 363);

✓ Control card of dispensary observation (onco) (form 030/u-onco, approved by the order of the Ministry of Health from 31.12.2020 № 363);

✓ Medical certificate of death (form No. 109)

§2.4 References and codifiers in the population cancert registry

Standardized coding systems are used in the SCR to compare the collected information. For some variables there are international coding systems that are mandatory for use, while others are coded based on local systems and requirements.

The most important international coding systems include:

✓ International Classification of Diseases 10th Revision (ICD-10)

✓ International Classification of Cancer Diseases 3rd Revision (ICD-O-3)

✓ TNM classification (latest revision)

✓ Clinical stage

In RUzb today, coding of oncological diseases (tumor topography) is done using ICD-10. In PCR, all MNs are registered with the code C00-C96 and in situ with the code D00-D09. If a patient has a primary-multiple tumor, each tumor is registered as a separate case and, accordingly, each MN case is also calculated by the software in the morbidity analysis.

Many other classifiers and directories are also used in coding variables (directory of place of residence, belonging to an ethnic group; sources of information about the place of treatment/diagnosis; surgeries, drugs, radiation therapy devices, laboratory tests (molecular-biological and genetic), etc.).

§ 2.5 Statistical processing of the obtained results

Data presentation and statistical analysis were performed in accordance with the requirements for biomedical research. Qualitative indicators are presented as absolute values and relative frequencies, 95% confidence intervals (CI) for the fraction or 95% CI for the difference of fractions. When comparing two indicators, the Z criterion was used [15].

A significance level of $p<0.05$ was adopted in the study. When deciding whether to reject the null hypothesis in favor of the alternative hypothesis, it was considered that the deviation of the calculated statistics from the corresponding distribution with a critical level of 0.05 and below was considered significant, and the null hypothesis was rejected. Otherwise, it was assumed that there were no sufficient statistical grounds for rejecting the null hypothesis.

CHAPTER III. DEMOGRAPHIC SITUATION AND CANCER MORBIDITY IN THE REPUBLIC OF UZBEKISTAN

§ 3.1 Demographic situation in the Republic of Uzbekistan

The average annual number of permanently residing population in RUzb in 2020 was 33,905,242, which is 650,300 more than in 2019.Rural residents accounted for 16,761,076 and urban residents 17,144,166, representing 49.4% and 50.6% respectively. It is worth noting that male population prevailed over female population with 17,045,288 (50.3%) and 16,859,954 (49.7%) respectively. The highest number of population was observed in Samarkand (3,877,355 - 11.4% share in the total population of the republic), Fergana (3,752,034 - 11.1%) and Kashkadarya (3,280,418 - 9.7%) oblasts, and the lowest in Syrdarya (846,260 - 2.5%), Navoi (997,100 - 2.9%) and Jizzak (1,382,060 - 4.1%) oblasts (Figure 3.1).

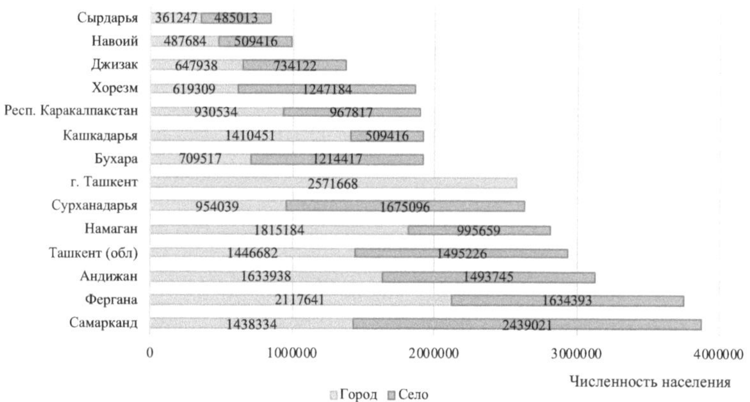

Fig. 3.1 Average annual number of urban and rural population by regions of the Republic of Uzbekistan

When considering the age structure of the population of RUzb, it is important to note that 33.6% of the population is aged 0-17 years and 43.5% is aged 18-44 years (Figure 3.2).

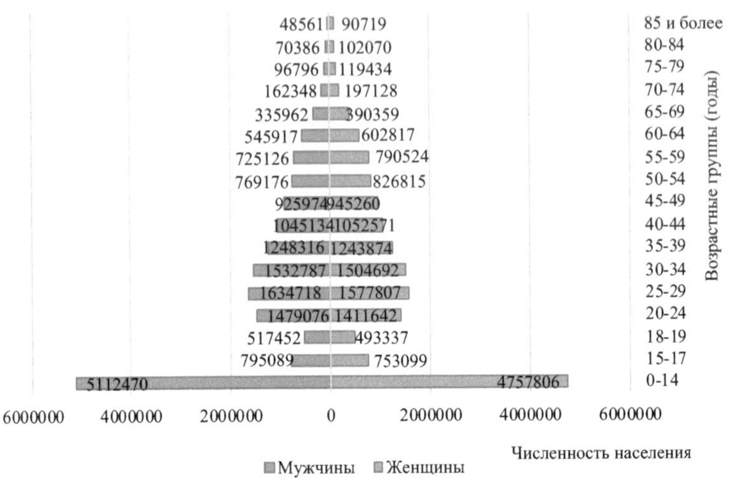

Fig. 3.2 Average annual population of the Republic of Uzbekistan by age and sex, 2020.

§ 3.2 Analysis of the morbidity rate of malignant neoplasms in the Republic of Uzbekistan

In 2020, 21,976 cases of MN were diagnosed for the first time in RUzb, including 9,059 cases diagnosed among men and 12,917 among women.

The crude intensive MN morbidity rate (per 100,000 population) was 64.8 *(*data of the State Statistics Committee of RUzb on the average annual population for 2020 were used to calculate all indicators*)*, which is 15.6% higher than in 2009. The highest ST incidence rates for 2020 were observed for breast (9.8 per 100,000 population), stomach (5.1) and cervical (4.8) (Figure 3.3).

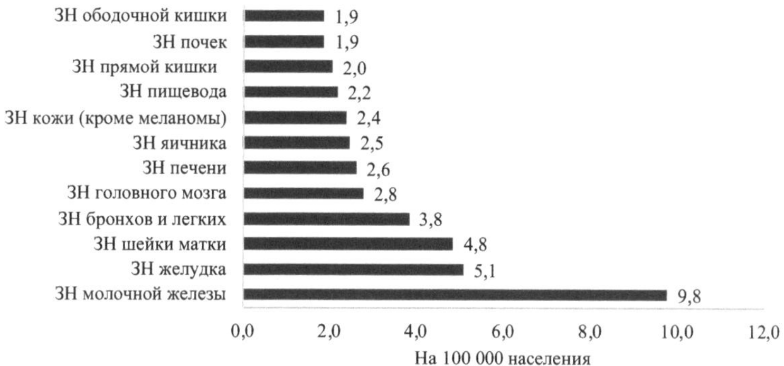

Fig. 3.3 Crude intensity indicators of malignant neoplasms morbidity in the Republic of Uzbekistan (per 100,000 population), 2020.

In the female population (Figure 3.4), the leading positions were MNs of the breast (19.5 per 100,000 female population), cervix (9.7), and ovary (4.9), while in the male population (Figure 3.5), the leading positions were of the stomach (6.2 per 100,000 male population), bronchi and lung (5.4), and prostate (3.0).

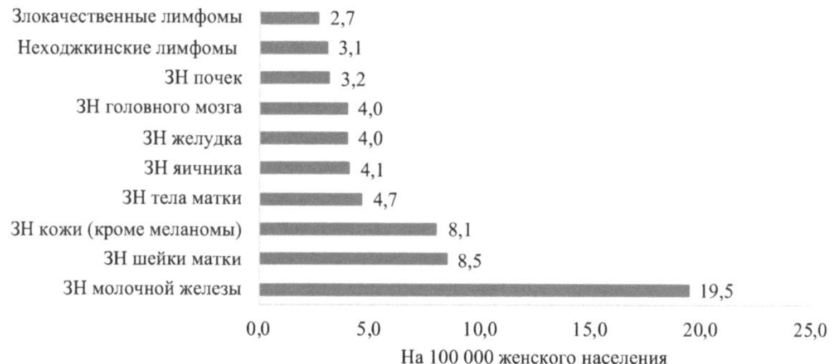

Fig. 3.4 Crude intensity-based incidence rates of malignant neoplasms in the female population of the Republic of Uzbekistan (per 100,000 population), 2020.

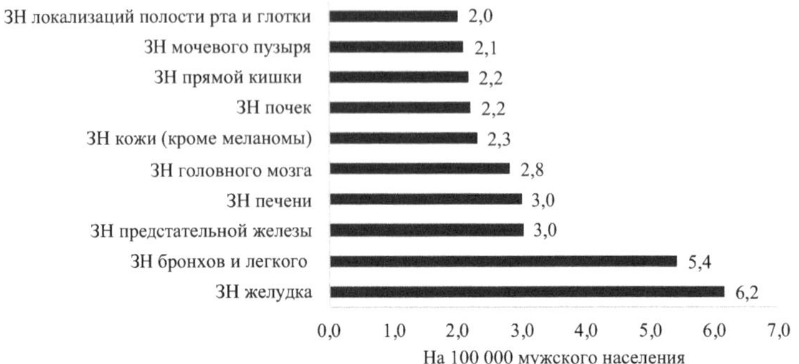

Fig. 3.5 Crude intensive incidence rates of malignant neoplasms in the male population of the Republic of Uzbekistan (per 100,000 population), 2020.

Analyzing the incidence rate among different age groups, it was noted that up to 70-74 years of age there was a dynamic increase in the rate (505.7 per 100,000 population). However, after 74 years of age there was a significant decrease in MN morbidity (Fig. 3.6).

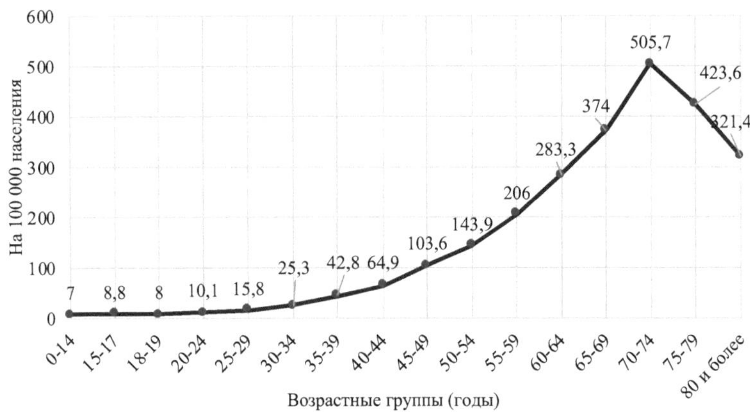

Fig. 3.6 Age-specific incidence rates of malignant neoplasms in the population of the Republic of Uzbekistan (per 100,000 population), 2020.

Analyzing the primary oncological morbidity among certain age groups, it was noted that in the age group up to 30 years old, hemoblastosis (26.4%), brain (16.3%), bone and joint (6.9%) and kidney (5.7%) MNs are registered quite often. In the 30-45 age group, the most frequently reported MNs were breast (23.5%), cervical (10.8%), and brain (8.8%). In patients aged 45-65 years, breast (18.2%), cervical (10.0%), stomach (7.6%), and lung (7.3%) MNs are more frequent. At the same time, among the older age group, the highest proportion of MNs occurred in the stomach (10.5%), lung (9.2%) and skin (8.3%).

It should be noted that in the morbidity structure of men in the age group 30-45 years, brain MNs (14.3%), lymphomas (13.6%), testicular MNs (10.0%) and stomach MNs (8.0%) prevail, while in women - breast MNs (34.3%), cervical MNs (15.9%), lymphomas (6.4%) and brain tumors (6.3%). There is a discrepancy in the structure of morbidity in the age group 45-65 years: in men, lung (13.5%), stomach (13.2%) and liver (6.0%) MNs are more frequently registered, in women - breast (29.5%), cervical (16.3%) and ovarian (6.7%) MNs. In the older age group, stomach (14.0%), lung (13.1%) and prostate (8.8%) MNs predominate in men, and breast (17.8%), skin (9.4%) and cervical (7.5%) MNs predominate in women.

§ 3.3 Characteristics of the organization of oncological care in Bukhara region

Bukhara oblast was selected to assess the quality of organization of oncological care in RUzb. Bukhara oblast consists of 11 rural districts and 2 cities. The population of Bukhara oblast at the end of 2020 amounted to 1,923,934, i.e. 5.7% of the total population of the republic. It should be emphasized that 82.3% of Bukhara oblast is made up of rural residents, and urban residents only 17.7%. The largest population size was in Bukhara city (303,348 - 15.8%), Gijduvan (280,187 - 14.6%) and Korakul

(176,914 - 9.2%) districts, the smallest - in Kogon (18,290 - 1.0%), Korovulbazar (61,124 - 3.2%) and Peshkin (78,040 - 4.1%) districts (Figure 3.7).

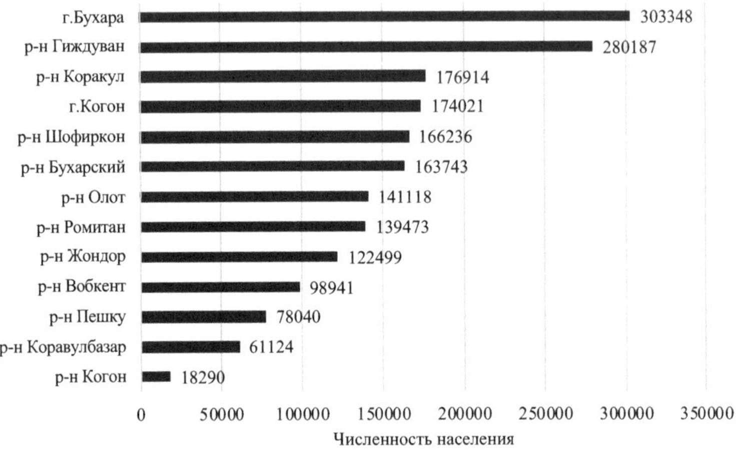

Fig. 3.7 Average annual population of Bukhara region, 2020.

Of the total population of Bukhara region, 963,523 (50.1%) are male and 960,411 (49.9%) are female (Figure 3.8). Studying the age category of the population of Bukhara region, it can be concluded that the majority of the population, as well as throughout the country, are children aged 0-17 years and young people aged 18-44 years, making up respectively 31.6% and 43.3% of the total population of Bukhara region.

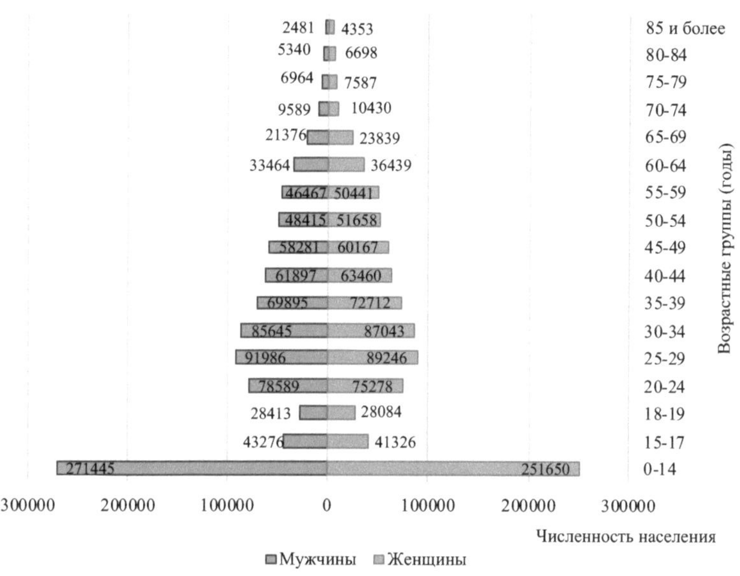

Fig. 3.8 Average annual population of Bukhara oblast by sex and age, 2020.

The number of oncology beds in Bukhara Oblast in 2020 was 143. From 2016 to 2020, the number of beds increased by 13, i.e. by 9.1%. In 2020, 6,834 patients were hospitalized in the Bukhara branch of the RSNPMCRC. The average length of stay of a patient in an oncology bed was 6.8 days. The average occupancy of an oncology bed was 344.2 days.

In 2020 in Bukhara region, the number of staff positions of doctors in the oncology branch was 90.5 of them employed was 90.5 (100%), and oncologists– 74.

Also in Bukhara oblast there are 15 oncologic offices in the districts of the oblast. Staff positions of district oncologists in Bukhara oblast are 20.5 rates, of which 17.25 are employed. Of the employed oncologists in the district polyclinics of Bukhara oblast (19 doctors), 90% of them have specialization in oncology (Table 3.1).

Table 3.1.

Information on district oncologists in Bukhara region, 2020.

Areas/cities Bukhara province	Oncologist's office (abs.num.)	Staffing of district oncologists		Individuals (absolute number)	Specialization
		allocated	employed		
Bukhara city	2	2,5	1,0	2	Surgeon Oncologist
Kogon	1	0,5	0,5	1	Oncologist
Olot district	1	1,25	1,25	1	Oncologist
Bukhara district	1	1,5	1,5	1	Surgeon
Vobkent district	1	1,5	1,5	2	Oncologist
Gijduvan district	2	3,0	3,0	2	Oncologist Oncologist
Kogon district	1	1,0	1,0	1	Oncologist
Korakul district	1	2,5	0,75	1	Oncologist
Koravul Bazaar district	1	0,25	0,25	1	ENT surgeon
Peshku district	1	1,5	1,5	2	Oncologist
Romitan district	1	1,75	1,75	1	Oncologist
Jondor district	1	2,25	2,25	3	Oncologist
Chauffircon district	1	1,0	1,0	1	Oncologist
Total	15	20,5	17,25	19	16/3

§ 3.3.1 Analysis of primary documentation of patients with malignant neoplasms in Bukhara oblast

Having analyzed outpatient records, case histories and extracts from primary medical documentation, a number of deficiencies in their completion were noted.

Despite the fact that the ICD-10 includes diseases with codes C00-C96 (C97 may be filled in additionally to indicate the number of patients suffering from primary-multiple MNs) and MNs in situ, i.e. ICD-10 codes D00-D09, in most of the analyzed documents patients with MNs in situ were not registered. There is often a tendency to fill in primary-multiple oncologic diseases (ICD-10 code C97) as a single disease without specifying the exact topography of each MN. It should be noted that each case of primary multiple cancers is registered as a separate case.

Also, the most common error is the presence of notifications when a patient is diagnosed with precancerous (obligate) disease (clinical group Ia and Ib).

Notices and extracts from the medical records of inpatients are written illegibly, with abbreviations of the patient's initials, date of birth, diagnosis and treatment. Moreover, the full clinical diagnosis is not always written (there is no precise indication of MN localization), in case of MN of one of the paired organs the side of the lesion is often not indicated, and in the presence of metastases the exact organ of the lesion is not indicated.

Quite often the stage of the disease according to the domestic classification (I-IV, stage not established) and clinical group (2-4) are not written, often only the TNM system stage is indicated. In the data on morphologic verification, the full text, the number of morphologic examination, the degree of differentiation and the date of the examination are not always written. This significantly complicates the process of registering patients and reduces the quality of the information obtained.

A number of errors in filling out death certificates for MN patients when determining the underlying cause of death have been identified.

Errors in removing MN patients from dispensary registration have been revealed. Thus, for basal cell skin cancer the mandatory dispensary observation is not more than 5 years, while in some districts/cities of Bukhara oblast patients with this disease are registered much longer.

§ 3.3.2 Study of the morbidity structure of malignant neoplasms in the population of Bukhara oblast

According to the data collected, 1,584 cases of MN were detected for the first time in Bukhara oblast in 2020: 715 (45.1%) among men and 869 (54.9%) among women. The crude intensive MN incidence rate per 100,000 population in Bukhara oblast in 2020 was 82.3.

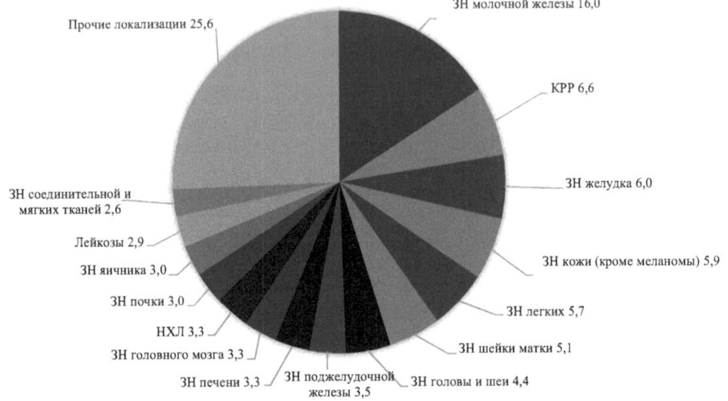

The leading positions in the structure of oncologic diseases of the population of Bukhara oblast were occupied by: breast (16.0%), colorectal (6.6%) and stomach (6.0%) diseases, Fig.3.9.

Fig.3.9 Structure of morbidity rate of malignant neoplasms in the population of Bukhara oblast, 2020.

The most frequent cancer pathologies among the female population in 2020 were breast (29.1%), cervical (9.2%) and ovarian (5.4%), while among the male population the most frequent were lung (9.5%); colorectal (9.0%) and stomach (8.7%), Figure 3.10.

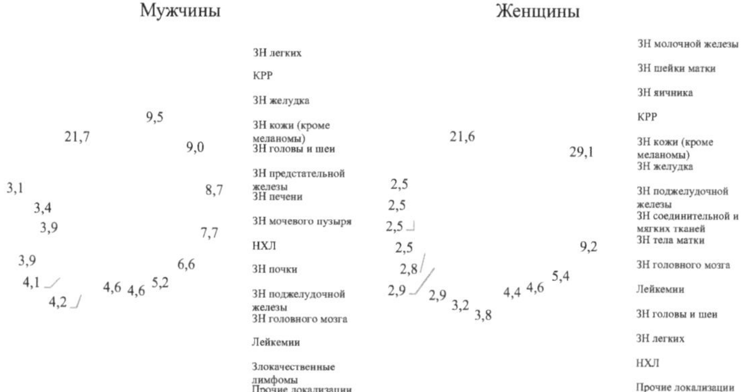

Fig.3.10 Structure of morbidity by malignant neoplasms of female and male population of Bukhara region (%), 2020.

Based on the data presented in Figure 3.10, the specific weight of colorectal cancer in women (4.6%) is almost 2 times lower than the same indicator (9.0%) in men ($p<0.05$). Moreover, the specific weight of lung MN in men (9.5%) is 3.8 times higher than in women (2.5), $p<0.05$. Also, the specific weight of MN of head and neck organs in men was 2.6 times ($p<0.05$) higher than in women.

Analyzing cancer morbidity by age (Fig. 3.11), it should be noted that a significant increase in this indicator begins with the age group of 45-49 years old, the peak incidence was observed among MN patients aged 75-79 years (577.3 per 100,000 population).

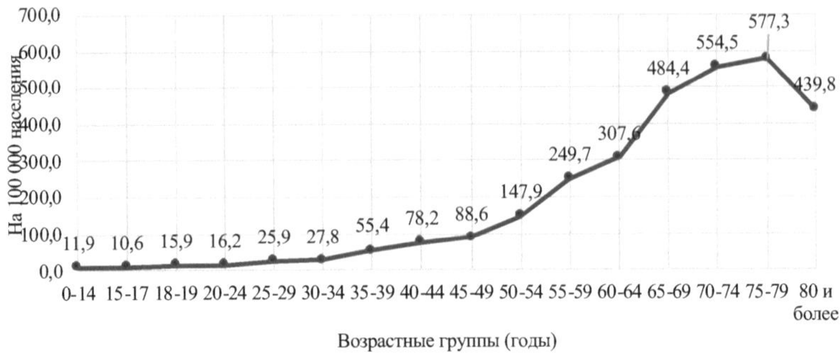

Fig.3.11 Age-specific incidence rates of malignant neoplasms in the population of Bukhara oblast (per 100,000 population of the corresponding age), 2020.

There is a tendency to increase the incidence of MN in men from 45-49 years of age, and in women - from 30-34 years of age. The peak of morbidity in men falls on the persons of old age - 80 years and older, in women - 75-79 years (Fig.3.12).

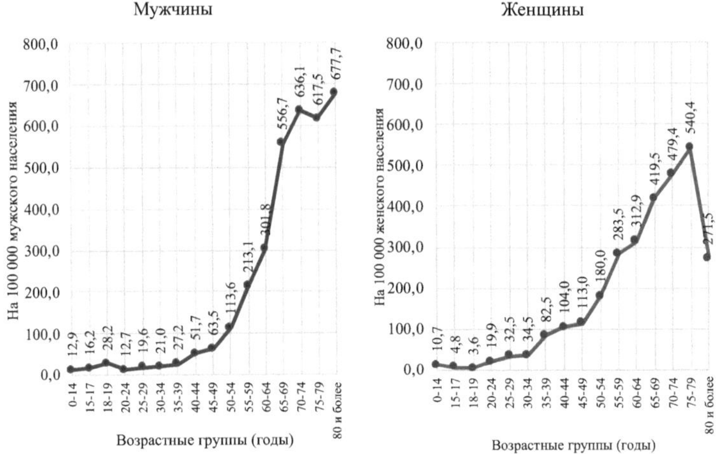

Fig.3.12 Age-specific incidence rates of malignant neoplasms among female and male population of Bukhara oblast (per 100,000 population of corresponding age), 2020.

Analyzing the structure of oncological morbidity among all first diagnosed MNs by age, it should be noted that in Bukhara oblast up to 30 years of age, hemoblastoses (31.6%), brain MNs (10.5%), bone and joint MNs (8.6%) prevailed. In the age group of 30-44 years - MN of breast (29,3%), lymphomas (9,8%) and brain (9,3%). In patients in the age group of 45-64 years, breast (19.9%), cervical (7.0%) and gastric (6.8%) MNs were frequently registered. At the same time, skin (11.9%), lung (10.1%), and breast (8.0%) MNs were more frequently registered among older patients, Figures 3.13-3.14.

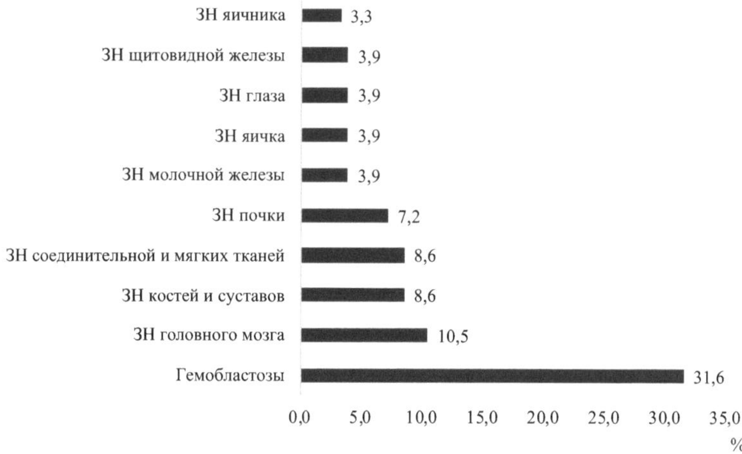

Fig.3.13 Structure of morbidity of malignant neoplasms in the population of Bukhara oblast under 30 years of age, %

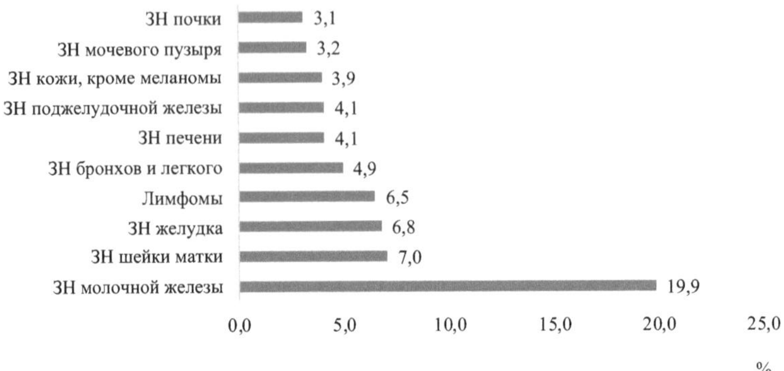

Fig.3.14 Structure of morbidity with malignant neoplasms of population of Bukhara region at the age of 45-64 years, %

In men and women under 30 years of age, hemoblastoses were most common, accounting for 39.7% and 23.0%, respectively. It should be noted that in men in the age group of 30-44 years brain MN (13.0%), lymphoma (13.0%) and thyroid MN (10.1%) prevailed; in women - breast MN (42.3%), cervical MN (9.6%) and lymphoma (8.3%), Fig. 3.15.

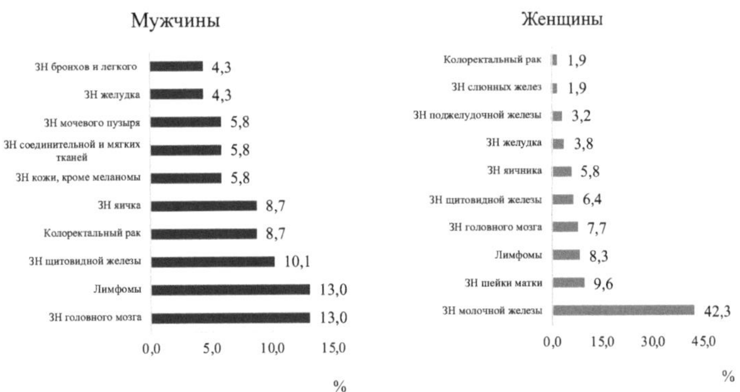

Fig.3.15 Structure of morbidity of malignant neoplasms in male and female population of Bukhara region at the age of 30-44 years, %

In men aged 45-64 years, gastric (11.0%), lung (8.9%) and lymphoma (8.2%) MNs were more common, while in women, breast

(33.7%), cervical (12.0%) and lymphoma (5.3%) MNs were more common, Figure 3.16.

Мужчины
ЗН почки 4,8
ЗН предстательной железы 4,8
ЗН кожи, кроме меланомы 4,8
ЗН поджелудочной железы 5,8
ЗН печени 6,5
ЗН мочевого пузыря 7,2
Колоректальный рак 7,5
Лимфомы 8,2
ЗН бронхов и легкого 8,9
ЗН желудка 11,0
0,0 5,0 10,0 15,0
%
Женщины
ЗН пищевода 2,4
ЗН поджелудочной железы 2,9
ЗН кожи, кроме меланомы 3,3
ЗН тела матки 3,8
ЗН желудка 3,8
ЗН яичника 4,8
Колоректальный рак 4,8
Лимфомы 5,3
ЗН шейки матки 12,0
ЗН молочной железы 33,7
0,0 10,0 20,0 30,0 40,0
%

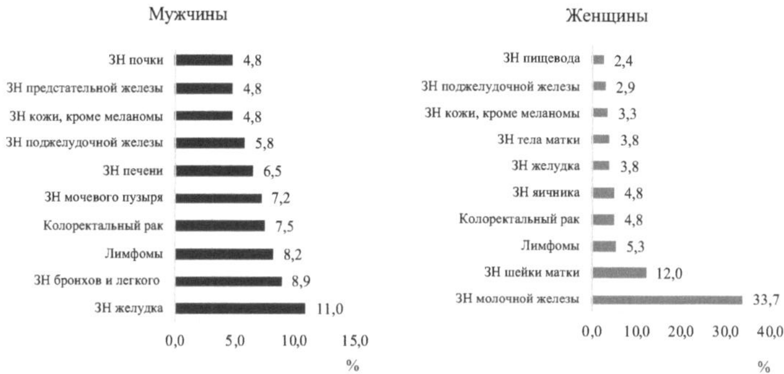

Fig.3.16 Structure of malignant neoplasms morbidity of male and female population of Bukhara region at the age of 45-64 years, %

In the age group of 65 years and older, MNs of the lung (13.8%), skin, except melanoma (13.4%) and colorectal zone (12.7%) were more frequently registered in men, while in women - MNs of the breast (18.1%), skin, except melanoma (10.0%) and colorectal zone (6.8%). It should be emphasized that rather high rates of skin neoplasms (i.e., 9.1% in men and 9.6% in women) and colorectal cancer (i.e., 13.1% in men and 7.2% in women) determine the focus of diagnostic measures in the older age group.

§ 3.3.3 Analysis of morbidity rate of malignant neoplasms by districts and cities of Bukhara oblast

Figure 3.17 shows the structure of ST morbidity in the population of districts and cities of Bukhara oblast. The highest specific weight fell on Bukhara city (18.4%), Gijduvan district (12.1%) and Zhondor district (9.6%), the lowest - on Kagan district (4.5%), Kagan city (4.0%) and Karaulbazar district (1.0%).

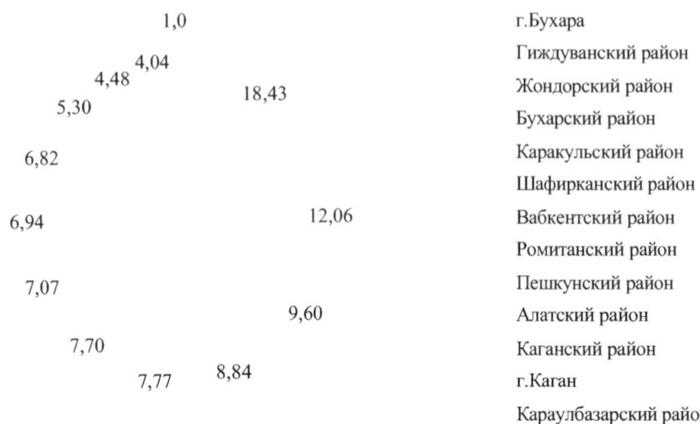

Fig.3.17 Structure of malignant neoplasm morbidity rate of districts/cities of Bukhara oblast (%), 2020.

The highest crude intensive MN incidence rates were found in Kagan city (104.7 per 100,000 inhabitants), Bukhara city (104.2) and Kagan district (91.0), while the lowest rates were found in Gijduvan (63.0), Shafirkan (69.0) and Karakul (75.1) districts (Figure 3.18).

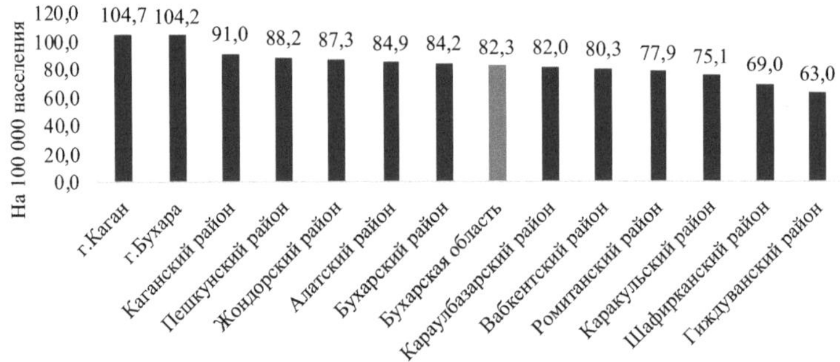

Fig.3.18 Crude intensity indicators (per 100,000 population) of malignant neoplasm morbidity in Bukhara oblast, 2020.

Analyzing the distribution of patients by age groups in Bukhara oblast (Table 3.2), it was revealed: the highest number of registered MN cases was observed at the age of 45-64 years (44.8%) and 65 years and more (31.4%), in total - 76.2%; at the age of 0-17 years - 4.5%, 18-30 years - 5.1%, 30-44 years - 14.2%.

A similar trend in the distribution of patients with MN was observed in districts and cities of Bukhara oblast. In the age group 45-64 years the specific weight ranged from 54.7% in Kagan city to 33.3% in Karaulbazar district. In the age group of 65 years and older, the highest number of patients with MN was observed in Karakul district (35.8%), and the lowest - in Karaulbazar district (20.0%). It should be noted that in Karaulbazar district the proportion of patients aged 30-44 years was 33.3%, which was the highest in this age group.

Table 3.2.

Specific weight (%) of first-time detected cases of malignant neoplasms by separate age groups of districts and cities of Bukhara region, 2020.

Neighborhood/city	Age breakdown, years (%):				
	0-17	18-29	30-44	45-64	65 +
Bukhara region	4,5	5,1	14,2	44,8	31,4
Bukhara city	3,8	2,7	10,3	47,3	36,0
Gijduvan district	5,2	3,7	16,2	43,5	31,4
Zhondor district	3,3	4,6	18,4	41,4	32,2
Bukhara district	4,3	5,7	12,9	44,3	32,9
Karakul district	4,9	8,1	11,4	39,8	35,8
Shafirkan district	6,6	9,0	17,2	46,7	20,5
Vabkent district	3,6	5,4	11,6	47,3	32,1
Romitan district	9,1	6,4	13,6	43,6	27,3
Peshkun district	5,6	5,6	20,4	38,0	30,6
Alat district	2,4	4,8	13,1	47,6	32,1
Kagan district	2,8	5,6	7,0	50,7	33,8
Kagan	0,0	3,1	18,8	54,7	23,4
Karaulbazar district	6,7	6,7	33,3	33,3	20,0

§ 3.3.4 Comparative analysis of standardized morbidity rates of malignant neoplasms among the population of Bukhara oblast

In the Republic of Uzbekistan to date, data comparison by regions of the country and the main localizations of MN is based on general - rough intensive indicators, which often leads to erroneous conclusions. Obtaining accurate estimates is possible with the help of standardized indicators, eliminating age composition in the compared groups. The composition (age distribution) of any of the groups being compared or their average composition, as well as the reference distribution obtained in other studies, can be taken as a standard. There are a variety of population standards used around the world, including the world standard, the European standard, the African standard, the truncated standard, and the SEER standard used in the United States. Also, it should be remembered that depending on the standard used, we get different levels of indicators, and when choosing a population standard, it is necessary to take into account the age composition of the population in the study population. There are three methods of standardization of indicators: direct, indirect and inverse, the choice of which depends on the goals, objectives and data set of the study [19, 20].

In this study, the direct method was used to calculate standardized morbidity rates, and the World (world) and African standards were taken as the standard (Table 3.3).

Table 3.3.

Different types of population standards

Age by year	Types of standard population distribution			
	World	truncated	European	African
0	2,400		1,600	2,000
1-4	9,600		6,400	8,000
5-9	10,000		7,000	10,000
10-14	9,000		7,000	10,000
15-19	9,000		7,000	10,000
20-24	8,000		7,000	10,000
25-29	8,000		7,000	10,000
30-34	6,000	6,000	7,000	10,000

35-39	6,000	6,000	7,000	10,000
40-44	6,000	6,000	7,000	5,000
45-49	6,000	6,000	7,000	5,000
50-54	5,000	5,000	7,000	3,000
55-59	4,000	4,000	6,000	2,000
60-64	4,000	4,000	5,000	2,000
65-69	3,000		4,000	1,000
70-74	2,000		3,000	1,000
75-79	1,000		2,000	0,500
80-84	0,500		1,000	0,300
85 and over	0,500		1,000	0,200
	100,0	31,000	100,000	100,0

As shown in Table 3.4, the standardized incidence rate calculated using the world standard (88.7±2.3 per 100,000 population) is slightly higher ($p>0.05$) than the crude intensive rate (82.3±4.1 per 100,000 population), while the incidence rate calculated using the African standard (56.7±1.5 per 100,000 population) is significantly lower ($p<0.001$). Significant variation of both standardized and crude intensive indicators by districts/cities of Bukhara oblast (African standard - from 46.0 to 64.8 per 100 000 population; World - from 68.1 to 99.7 per 100 000 population; crude intensive - from 63.0 to 104.7 per 100 000 population) and rather large standard errors of indicators are the evidence of errors in recording of primary MN morbidity.

Table 3.4.

Crude and standardized incidence rates of malignant neoplasms by districts/cities of Bukhara province, 2020.

Neighborhood/city	Crude figure			Standardized measure (World)			Standardized measure (African)		
	total	husband	wives	total	husband	wives	total	husband	wives
Bukhara region	82,3	74,2	90,5	88,7	87,0	91,1	56,7	51,8	61,8
Bukhara city	104,2	90,5	117,7	99,6	99,8	100,0	60,4	55,2	65,7
Gijduvan district	63,0	51,6	74,8	73,3	65,7	80,9	46,0	39,9	52,2

Zhondor district	87,3	74,4	100,0	97,3	91,5	103,2	64,0	54,7	73,1
Bukhara district	84,2	77,9	90,6	92,9	89,2	97,1	57,2	51,5	63,0
Karakulsky district	75,1	70,5	79,7	92,7	94,5	91,7	57,7	57,1	58,4
Shafirkan district	69,0	56,1	82,1	68,1	55,2	81,7	49,4	37,8	61,2
Vabkent district	80,3	79,9	80,7	90,7	99,8	88,4	57,6	59,7	58,8
Romitan district	77,9	51,7	104,9	87,8	65,2	112,1	57,4	37,0	78,8
Peshkun district	88,2	84,8	91,5	99,2	101,8	97,4	64,7	65,2	64,6
Alat district	84,9	80,7	89,1	96,5	98,0	95,2	60,4	57,9	62,9
Kagan district	91,0	116,6	65,9	99,7	137,3	67,5	57,7	77,3	40,7
Kagan	104,7	114,2	95,7	94,8	111,3	82,4	64,8	65,9	65,4
Karaulbazar district	82,0	99,3	65,0	79,1	113,0	47,8	62,3	70,6	53,1

Crude intensive incidence rate per 100,000 male population of Bukhara oblast was 74.2+2.8 (95% CI: 68.8÷79.6), standardized rate (World and African) - 87.0+8.4 (95% CI: 70.3÷103.6) and 51.8+2.1 (95% CI: 43.3÷60.3). In the female population: crude intensive rate was 90.5+3.1 per 100,000 population (95% CI: 84.5÷96.5), World standard was 91.1+6.8 (95% CI: 77.7÷104.6) and African standard was 61.8+2.3 (95% CI: 54.2÷69.3).

It is worth noting that the Central Asian states are now in a state of demographic revolution, which is characterized by a high birth rate and, consequently, an increase in the proportion of persons aged 0-17 years in the age structure of the population [17]. Thus, the use of any of the currently existing population standards will give overestimates or underestimates of morbidity levels, which should be taken into account when conducting epidemiological studies.

§ 3.3.5 Analysis of the formation of stages of primary cases of malignant neoplasms in the population of Bukhara oblast

TNM classification for malignant tumors was first proposed by P. Denoix in 1943-1952. Already in 1958, the International Union Against

Cancer (UICC) issued the first recommendations on TNM classification of breast and larynx MNs, and in 1978 - the first edition of TNM classification for all MNs. Subsequently, this classification has been revised many times, and the latest current version is TNM classification of the 8th revision, and for some nosological forms - 9th revision.

TNM and clinical stage, which were established at the time of confirmed diagnosis, do not change regardless of the regression/progression of the tumor process. TNM and clinical stage are collected for each MN localization in a tabular form. It should be noted that clinical stage is one of the main factors that determines the choice of tactics and type of treatment.

There is also a pathologic classification - pTNM, which is based on the results of surgical treatment and histologic examination. The use of pTNM allows for a more accurate determination of MN disease stage [2, 37, 59].

To assess the correspondence between TNM and clinical stages, the primary documentation of 824 patients suffering from MN (the most frequent in the structure of cancer morbidity in Bukhara region, Table 3.5) was analyzed. The standards of diagnostics and treatment of malignant neoplasms in Uzbekistan, Russian Federation, Republic of Belarus, ESMO and NCCN, where the 8th edition of TNM of MNs is indicated, were taken as a basis [37].

Table 3.5.

General structure of malignant neoplasm morbidity of the population of Bukhara region, 2020.

Localization of MN	First-time detected cases	%
Mammary gland	253	16,0
Colorectal cancer	104	6,6

Stomach	95	6,0
Skin (except melanoma)	93	5,9
Light	90	5,7
Cervix	80	5,1
Pancreas	56	3,5
Liver	53	3,3
Others	760	48,0
Total:	1584	100,0

Having analyzed 824 cases of first registered MNs in Bukhara oblast, it was revealed that in 96 (11.7%) cases the stage was incorrectly determined. It should be emphasized that the most discrepancies were observed in the staging of pancreatic MN (32.1%), colorectal cancer (18.3%) and liver MN (15.1%), Table 3.6. The most frequent error (46.9%) in establishing the clinical stage of the disease was the use of the numerical value of T category (TNM classification) as an indicator of stage.

Table 3.6.

Number of mismatches between TNM and clinical stages of individual localizations of malignant neoplasms, Bukhara region, 2020.

Localization	Mismatch between TNM and clinical stages (abs.num.)	% of first-time cases
Mammary gland	14	5,5
Colorectal cancer	19	18,3
Stomach	13	13,7
Skin (except melanoma)	10	10,8
Light	10	11,1
Cervix	4	5,0
Pancreas	18	32,1
Liver	8	15,1
Total errors	96	11,7

Studying inconsistencies in clinical stage staging in Bukhara oblast, we can conclude that the majority of errors were in stage III (54.2%) and II (31.3%). That is, instead of stage II and IV, stage III was diagnosed in 40.6% and 12.5% of cases. The same situation with stage II, instead of stage III and IV, stage II was diagnosed in 18.8% and 5.2% of cases (Table 3.7).

Table 3.7.

Number of mismatches between TNM and clinical stages of malignant neoplasm cases in the population of Bukhara region, 2020.

Stage corrected	Primary stage	TNM and clinical stage mismatch (abs.num.)	%
I	II	7	7,3
	III	1	1,0
II	I	3	3,1
	III	39	40,6
III	II	18	18,8
	IV	11	11,5
IV	II	5	5,2
	III	12	12,5
Total:		96	100,0

Considering clinical and TNM stages by districts/cities of Bukhara region, it was noted that the highest proportion of mismatches was in: Bukhara city (20.8%), Gijduvan (13.5%), Zhondor (12.5%), Bukhara (11.5%) and Shafirkan (9.4%) districts - a total of 67.7% of all mismatches (Figure 3.19).

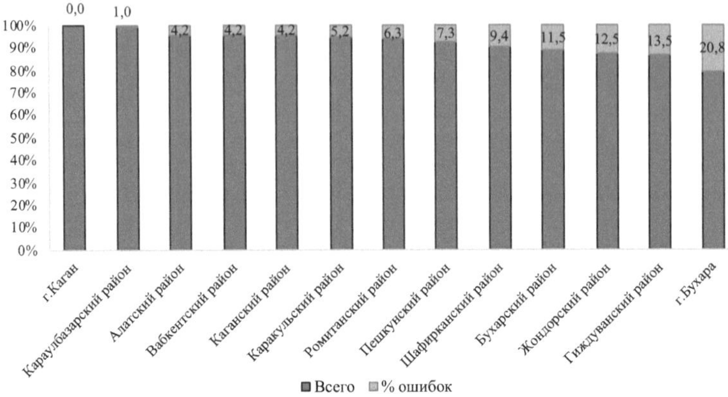

Figure 3.19 Percentage of disease stage mismatch in districts/cities of Bukhara province, 2020.

Summary

Analysis of the organization of oncology service in Bukhara region has shown that despite 100% employment of oncology posts in the branch of RSNPMCHC&R there is a shortage of oncology specialists in the district offices. The incidence of MN in Bukhara oblast was 82.3 per 100,000 population. The leading positions in the structure of cancer morbidity were occupied by breast, colorectal and stomach diseases. There are also some differences in the structure of morbidity in different age groups: in the age group up to 30 years of age hemoblastosis, MN of the brain and bones, joints are more characteristic, at the age of 30-44 years - MN of the breast, lymphoma and brain, and in older age - MN of the skin, lung and breast.

The analysis of primary documentation indicates a number of deficiencies in filling out discharge summaries, notifications and neglect protocols, namely: coding of diagnosis (ICD-10), stages of disease (both clinical and TNM), clinical group.

Correct staging plays an important role in the selection of treatment methods. Based on the analysis of the presented data, we can conclude that in 11.7% of cases the treatment tactics could have been selected incorrectly. An important role in determining further treatment is played by pTNM, which cannot be analyzed due to the absence of a population-based cancer registry. In addition, the staging of the disease according to the generally accepted clinical classification (I-IV) in Bukhara region occurs without letter specification (Ia-c, IIa-c, etc.), which also plays an important role in the choice of appropriate treatment.

Comparative analysis of standardized indicators of MN morbidity in Bukhara oblast showed that when using the world standard, the standardized indicator is slightly higher than the crude intensive indicator, while the morbidity indicator calculated according to the African standard is significantly lower than the crude intensive one. Significant variation in both standardized and crude intensive rates, as well as rather large standard errors of the rates, indicate some inaccuracies in the available MN registration system. In the absence of the Kancer register and the presence of errors in the registration of primary MN cases, it is justified to use standardized indicators (World standard) to assess the oncoepidemiological situation in the country, as well as in the comparative analysis of morbidity rates with other countries of the world.

CHAPTER IV. METHODOLOGICAL ASPECTS TO THE POPULATION CANZER-REGISTER

The main purpose of the PCR in RUzb is to keep personalized records with regular follow-up of a patient with MN, as well as to keep records of first diagnosed cases of MN, and to keep information about the treatment provided.

The objectives of the RCR also include:

1. Registration of MN cases and their further completion, i.e. information on treatment - correct adherence to standards and protocols of treatment, diagnostics - correct diagnosis and dispensary. Quality control of the entered data.
2. Researching and conducting analysis of available data followed by the preparation of various reports.
3. Generalization of information in the RPC for the formation of state statistics for subsequent submission to the Ministry of Health.
4. Formation of annual analytical statistical compilations of the oncology service.
5. Conducting scientific, epidemiological, and government research programs that are necessary to improve cancer care in the country.
6. Protect and maintain existing and retrospective data in the SCR.
7. Opportunities for international scientific research.

The basic part of the RUzb RCT is the offices of district oncologists of RMOs/GMOs. Personal data on MN cases are sent from the district oncologist's office to the regional branches of the RNNPMCHC&R.

In the regional branches of RSPMCoIR the RWC RUzb functions in the form of register branches, on the basis of organizational and methodological departments.

At the republican level, the RUzb RPC, in its turn, represents a branch of the Cancer Prevention Center, which is a part of the Cancer Prevention Center. This department is engaged in monitoring the activity of regional cancer registries, forming and submitting reports to the Ministry of Health of RUzb, assessing the state of oncology service, planning anticancer activities in the regions and in the republic as a whole, assessing the oncoepidemiologic situation in each region, planning the purchase of expensive drugs and medical equipment, regular training seminars for medical personnel on international requirements for registration and registration of oncologists. Based on this, the structure of the RPC was developed.

§ 4.1 Structure of the population canzer-register

There are 5 main sections in the PKR system:

- Search - section for searching for a patient in the card index according to the specified parameters.
- New Patient - section for creating a card for a new patient
- Lists - section for viewing and creating patient lists and working with drafts.
- Statistics - section for the construction of state statistical and arbitrary statistical reporting in accordance with international requirements.
- Administration - section for managing the PKP system (user accounts, rights and roles).

§4.2 Searching by section

The registry system implements the ability to Search the following sections:

- ✓ Search by full name
- ✓ Information search
- ✓ Regulated search

*Additional lists to analyze in the database (*depending on the role, additional types of regulated searches may be available to analyze in the database):

- ✓ Mistaken patronymic
- ✓ Incomplete date of birth
- ✓ Incomplete m/w at the time of diagnosis
- ✓ The figure in the text of the operation

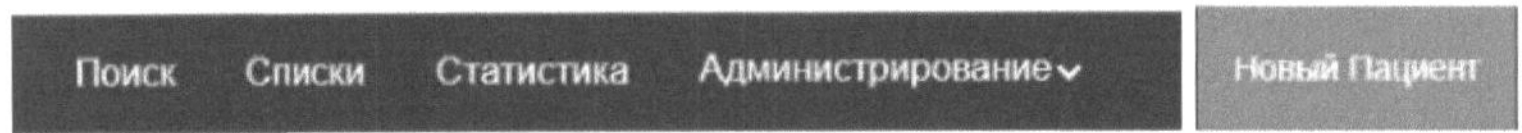

For the convenience of users, two options are implemented for searching and entering information into the RPC:

-Fields without any buttons (e.g. Surname, First Name, Patronymic, Outpatient Card No.) are for manual data entry.

Фамилия Имя Отчество

-Button fields imply both manual data entry and selection of a variant from the drop-down list and selection from the system directories.

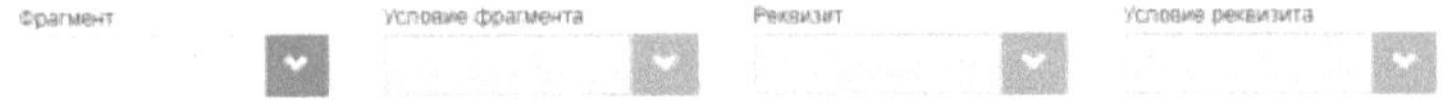

§ 4.3 Creating a new patient

Any cancer patient record in the PCP database consists of the following sections:

1. Passport part
2. Diagnoses
3. Treatment
4. Recurrences and metastases
5. Information on neglect
6. Clinical groups
7. Notes on medical examinations

Passport part

In the Passport section, basic personal and demographic information about the patient is entered. It is worth noting that the system has mandatory and optional fields, with the former marked with an "*":

I. Identification

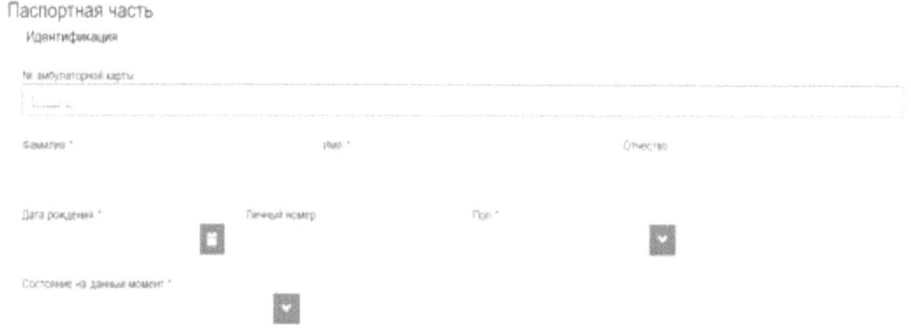

- ✓ Field - No. of outpatient card
- ✓ Field - Last Name *
- ✓ Field - Name *
- ✓ Field - Patronymic
- ✓ Field - Date of Birth *(dd.mm.yyyyyy)
- ✓ Field - PINFL *
- ✓ Field - Gender * (male/female)
- ✓ Field - Current status (Alive/Dead from complications of treatment/Dead from underlying disease/Departed/Diagnosis not confirmed/Discontinued due to expiration of observation period)

II. Place of residence

- ✓ Field - Resident* (city/village);
- ✓ Field - SOATO code * (System of designation of administrative-territorial object);
- ✓ Field - Mahalla / street / avenue / block / alley* (selected by SOATO classifier list);

- ✓ Field - Home
- ✓ Field - Corpus
- ✓ Field - Apartment
- ✓ Field - Postal code
- ✓ Field - Phone Numbers *
- ✓ Field - Email

III. Other information

- ✓ Field - Ethnic group / Nationality *
- ✓ Field - Education (basic/secondary/higher education)
- ✓ Field - Profession (directory of registered professions in the Republic of Uzbekistan)
- ✓ Field - Nationality
- ✓ Field - Date of enrollment* (dd.mm.yyyyy)
- ✓ Field - RMO/HMO (directory of medical institutions registered in the Republic of Uzbekistan)
- ✓ Field - Disability group (1, 2, 3, disabled child)
- ✓ Field - Dispensary registered in another RMO/GMO (registered for the first time/registered in another RMO/GMO)

IV. Information on attrition (death)

- ✓ Field - Disposal date* (dd.mm.yyyyy)
- ✓ Field - Source of information on disposal* (local classifier)
- ✓ Field - Where departed (directory of medical institutions registered in the Republic of Uzbekistan, CIS countries, near and far abroad)
- ✓ Field - Cause of Death (full ICD-10 reference)
- ✓ Field - Presence of tampering (yes/no)

Diagnoses

In the "Diagnoses" section, information about the patient's diagnoses and the dates of their establishment is entered. If several tumors (synchronous, metachronous) are detected in the patient, information about each diagnosis is entered separately:

- ✓ Field - ICD-10* Code (ICD-10 reference C00-C96, D00-D09)
- ✓ Field - Date of diagnosis* (dd.mm.yyyyy)
- ✓ Field - Date the diagnosis was canceled (dd.mm.yyyyyy)
- ✓ Field - Pairing indication (None/Left/Right/Obi-Organs/Unknown)
- ✓ Field - Pregnancy at diagnosis (yes/no)
- ✓ Field - Sources of information on diagnosis (list main forms)
- ✓ Field - Where information came from (directory of medical institutions registered in the Republic of Uzbekistan)
- ✓ Field - Place of residence at the time of diagnosis (SOATO - System of designation of administrative-territorial object)
- ✓ Field - Stage* (0, I, II, III, IV, not specified)
- ✓ Field - Final stage (after a full examination within 3 months)
- ✓ Field - Stage Refinement (a, b, c, d, E, S)
- ✓ Field - cT (TNM Classification 8th revision, 2017)
- ✓ Field - cN (TNM Classification 8th revision, 2017)
- ✓ Field - cM (TNM Classification 8th revision, 2017)
- ✓ Field - pT (TNM Classification 8th revision, 2017)
- ✓ Field - pN (TNM Classification 8th revision, 2017)
- ✓ Field - rM (TNM Classification 8th revision, 2017)
- ✓ Field - Plurality* (Major/Non-Major)
- ✓ Field - Conditions of detection* (Self-reported/ Detected in Onco-Nazorat office/ During other types of professional examinations/ During parallel professional examinations/ During screening/ Recorded posthumously with a diagnosis established during life/ Recorded posthumously without autopsy/ Recorded posthumously after autopsy).

✓ Field - Confirmation Method* (Histologic/ Cytologic - Hematologic/ Endoscopic/ Radiologic/ Clinical Only/ Isotopic/ Ultrasound/ Oncomarkers/ Myelogram)

✓ Field - ICD-O-3 Morphology (ICD-O-3 Morphology Guide)

✓ Field - Degree of differentiation * (High/Medium/Low/Undifferentiated/ T-cell/B-cell/0-cell/NK/cell/unknown)

✓ Field - Date of morphologic examination (dd.mm.yyyyy)

✓ The Diagnoses section contains fragments: General information about the diagnosis, data about the performed investigations (IHC specific/nonspecific, molecular genetic), Recurrences and metastases, Information about neglect and Physician consiliums.

✓ Field - ICD-O-3 morphology final, after surgery (ICD-O-3 morphology guide)

✓ Field - Degree of differentiation final, after surgery* (High/Medium/Low/Undifferentiated/ T-cell/B-cell/0-cell/NK/cell/unknown)

✓ Field - Date of morphologic examination final, after surgical intervention (dd.mm.yyyyy)

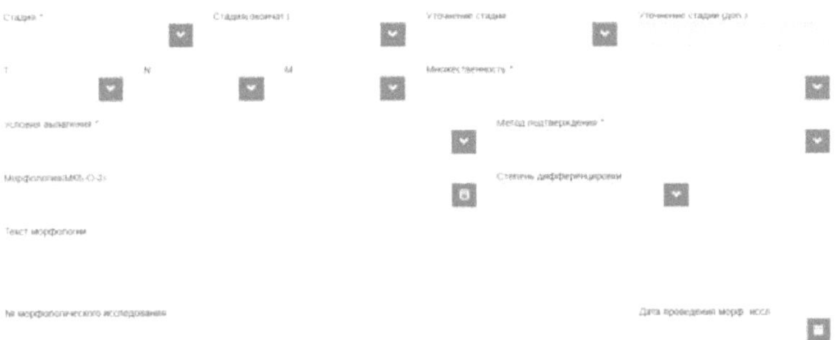

Immunohistochemical (IHC) findings.

This section presents the results of specific and nonspecific IHC tests. Specific GCIs include estrogen, progesterone, HER2 neu, Ki 67, PD-L1.

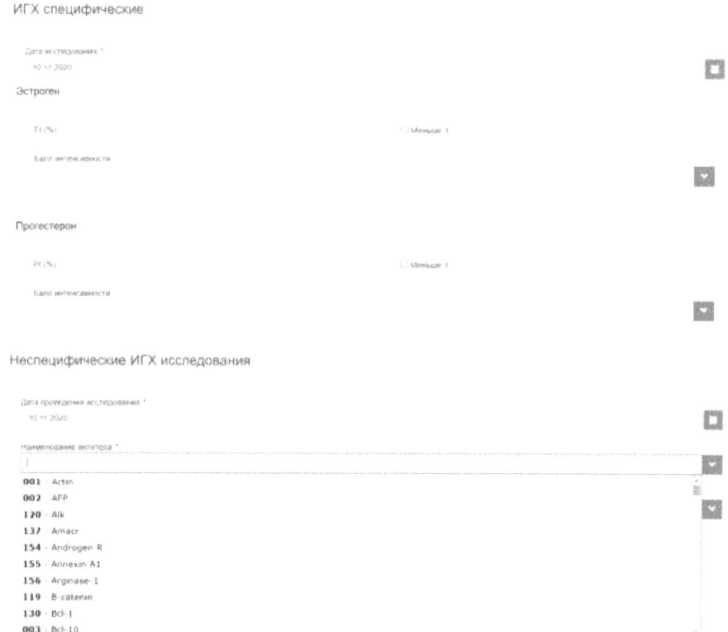

Results of molecular genetic studies.

In case of molecular genetic studies, the following fields shall be filled in:

- ✓ Field - Date of the study* (dd.mm.yyyyy)
- ✓ Study method (FISH/ Sequencing/ PCR/ Fragment analysis/ unknown)
- ✓ Variant of genetic disorder (Mutation / Amplification / Co-deletion / Translocation / Reassortment / Unknown)
- ✓ Result (detected/not detected)
- ✓ Gene (assay)

Archive

Subsections of the archive allow to keep records in case of changes in the patient's name, address, branch, as well as to track patient's calls to the branch, the archive of outpatient records

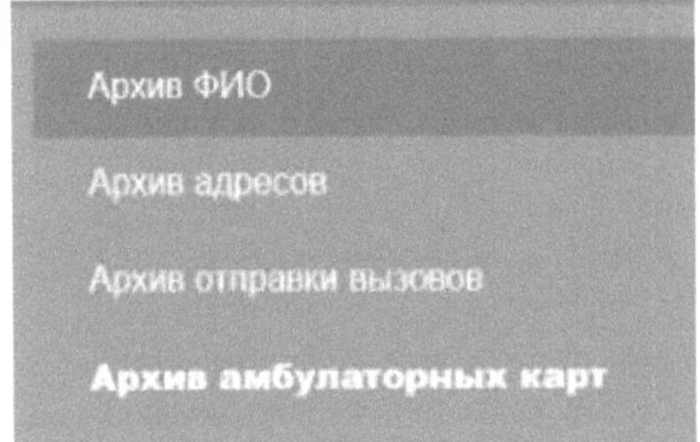

Treatment

The "Treatment" section is intended for entering information about the treatment carried out according to the diagnosis(s).

Several types and nature of treatment may be performed for a single diagnosis.

Note: Treatment courses may overlap if one treatment is inpatient and the other is outpatient. However, 2 inpatient courses of treatment cannot overlap.

Each treatment fragment is completed in a separate section - General Treatment Information:

Field - Treatment start date* (dd.mm.yyyyyy)

Field - Treatment Completion Date (dd.mm.yyyyyy)

Field - Treatment information (No information/Treated as an outpatient/Inpatient)

Field - Nature of treatment * (None/ Radical/ Palliative/ Symptomatic/ Rehabilitation/ Radical Incomplete/ Prophylactic/ Investigation/ For other diseases/ For complications)

Field - Type of special treatment * (Not performed/Surgical/ Distant radiation therapy/ Short-focus radiotherapy/ Short-focus radiotherapy/Combined radiotherapy: Cont.+ distant/ Combined radiotherapy: Cont.+ X-ray/ Chemotherapy (hormonal)/ Surgical+distance radiotherapy/Surgical+short-focus radiotherapy/ Surgical+short-focus radiotherapy/ Surgical+combined radiotherapy/ Surgical+contact radiotherapy/ Surgical+chemotherapy (hormonal).X-ray therapy/Surgery+combined radiotherapy/Surgery+contact radiotherapy/Surgery+chemotherapy (hormone therapy)/Complex chemoradiotherapy/ Surgery+radiation+radiation+chemotherapy (hormone therapy)/Radiopharmaceuticals/Contact radiation therapy/Other types of treatment/Surgery+radiopharmaceuticals/Combined radiation therapy:Remote Radiation Therapy+Radiation Therapy)

Field - Type of health care organization (with/without cancer centers)

Field - Place of treatment (place of treatment according to the directory of medical institutions RUzb)

Field - Reason for incomplete treatment (Patient refusal of special treatment/ Contraindication to special treatment/ Incurable patient/ Dynamic observation/ Active observation)

Surgical treatment

Information about each surgical intervention: nature of surgery, date of surgery and coding of surgery (according to the directory of surgical interventions for cancer patients) is mandatory.

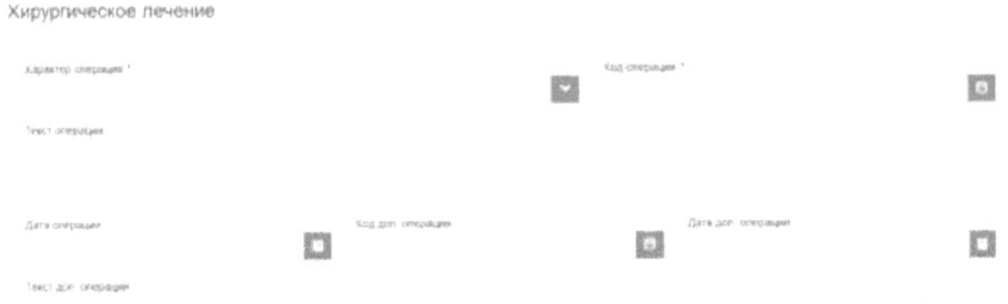

Chemotherapy treatment

All drugs used in chemotherapy treatment in RUzb are entered into the database in accordance with the approved drug reference book. In addition, the fields are filled in: Total drug dose, Unit of measurement, Method of administration and Date of administration.

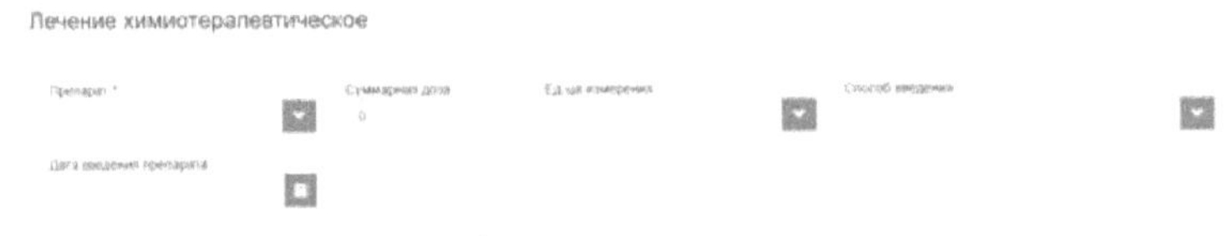

Radiation treatment (machines)

In Radiation treatment (devices) - mandatory details are filled in: Nature, Exposure Type, Exposure Zone and Total Dose. Additional details in this section are: Modifier, Organ, Single dose and Equivalent dose.

When filling in the "Nature*" field, it is necessary to select the nature of radiation exposure from the reference list: Preoperative / Intraoperative / Postoperative / Self-operative radical / Self-operative palliative / Self-operative symptomatic / Pre- and postoperative / Prophylactic (anti-rejection).

The field "Type of exposure*" is filled in according to the used radiation exposure: Remote / Radiotherapy / Intracavitary / Intrathecal / Intrathecal / Application / Intraluminal.

In the field "Area of exposure*" indicates what the irradiation is aimed at: Main focus / Regional MTS / Remote MTS / Main focus + areas of regional MTS / Main focus + areas of regional MTS + areas of remote MTS / Possible remote MTS.

When filling in the "Modifiers" field, it is necessary to indicate which modifier was used: Radioprotectors / Radiosensitizers / Local microwave hyperthermia / Barotherapy / General hyperthermia + artificial hyperglycemia + polychemotherapy.

The "Organ" field is filled in to specify the irradiation area of distant MTS: Lymph nodes / Bones / Liver / Lung (pleura) / Brain / Ovary / M/tissues / Adrenal gland / Other organs / Peritoneum.

Radiation treatment (radiopharmaceuticals)

When treating the patient with radiopharmaceuticals, the "Radiopharmaceutical*" field should be filled in: Brom-82 * Gallium-67 / Gallium-52 / Iron-59 / Gold-198 / Indium-111 / Iridium-192 / Ytterbium-169 / Yttrium-90,91 / Iodine-113 / Iodine-125 / Iodine-131 / Potassium-42 / Potassium-43 / Calcium-47 / Cobalt-58 / Cobalt-60 / Xenon-133 / Copper-64 / Metastrone / Sodium-24 / Mercury-197 / Ruthenium-106 / Selenium-75 / Strontium-85 / Strontium-87M / Strontium-89 / Strontium-90 / Technetium-99M / Tritium / Phosphorus-32 / Fluorine-18 / Chromium-61 / Cesium-137. The "Date of drug administration" field (dd.mm.yyyyy) and the "Dose" field (Gbc) are also filled in.

Other impacts

Other treatments include: Hyperthermia / Hyperglycemia / Magnetotherapy / Photodynamic therapy / Radiofrequency Oblation (RFA) / Local chemotherapy / Laser exposure (TTT) / Electrocoagulation

/ Electrochemical lysis / Microwave ablation (MVA) / Intravenous laser blood irradiation (ILBI) / Dendritic cell injection / BMC Mirena / CAR-T therapy / Blood replacement therapy.

The selected exposure type is entered in the "Type of exposure*" field and the "Start date of exposure" (dd.mm.yyyyy) and "End date of exposure" (dd.mm.yyyyy) fields are filled in.

Recurrences and metastases

The "Recurrences and metastases" section is intended for entering relevant data for each detection of disease recurrence or metastases (disease progression). When filling in the "Occurred process*" field, it is necessary to specify which process was registered: Recurrence / Regional metastases / Distant metastases / Biochemical recurrence / Process progression / Local spread process / Transformation. In case of regional or distant metastases it is necessary to fill in the field "Area of lesion": Lymph nodes / Bone / Liver / Lung (pleura) / Brain / Ovary / Soft tissue / Adrenal gland / Other organs / Peritoneum.

Information on neglect

The section "Information on neglect" is intended for entering the relevant data when the patient is diagnosed with stage III-IV disease of visually accessible localizations and stage IV of all MNs.

The "Date of first signs" field (dd.mm.yyyyy) is filled in from the anamnesis data. In the field "Cause of neglect" the main reason why the disease was detected in a neglected form is indicated, after reviewing each case at a medical conference and completing the appropriate protocol: Incomplete examination of the patient / Error in clinical diagnosis / Error in radiological diagnosis / Error in cyto-morphological diagnosis / Prolonged examination of the patient / Hidden course of the disease / Untimely application of the patient for help / Patient's refusal to be examined / Errors in dispensaryization of patients with chronic pathology / The protocol was not sorted out at the medical conference.

In the field "Reason for late diagnosis*" enter the main reason, which was determined at the medical conference, taking into account what category the patient belongs to according to the classes of dispensary, frequency of visits to primary health care facilities (with/without complaints), etc..: Persons subject to medical examinations. Violation of the terms of dispensary / Persons subject to medical examinations. Incomplete examination / Persons subject to medical examinations. Diagnostic error / Patients (benign diseases, pre-cancer). Violation of the terms of medical examination / Patients (Benign diseases, precancer). Incomplete examination / Patients (Benign diseases, precancer). Diagnostic error / Appeal with complaints. No examination was performed / Referral. Incomplete examination / Complaint. Diagnostic error / Referral without complaints. The examination was not carried out / Appeal without complaints. Incomplete examination / Appeal without complaints. Diagnostic error / Patient's refusal of examination / Rapidly progressive form of neoplasm / The protocol is not resolved.

Note: The additional block Information about referrals to other health care organizations appears when you specify information about neglect.

Clinical groups

The Clinical Groups section contains information about the patient's clinical groups (2, 3, 4). When transferring a patient from one clinical group to another, this section must always be filled in.

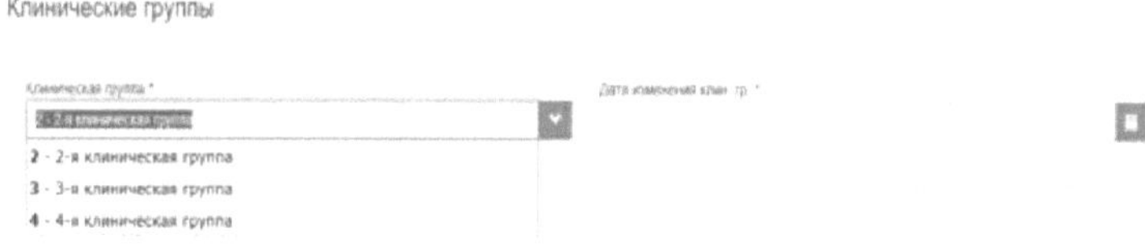

Notes on medical examinations

The "Dispensary notes" section can be automatically filled after adding treatment, if the value in the Treatment information field is Outpatient or Inpatient and the date of adding treatment is greater than the date of the last dispensary note. If the patient's appearance was marked or his/her fate was specified after the last course of treatment - the dispensary mark is filled in manually:

Field - Date of last contact* (dd.mm.yyyyyy)

Field - Contact note (Patient's refusal to come to the branch / Reported to the branch for a check-up / Received information from the medical institution at the place of residence / Reported to the medical institution for a check-up by a visiting team / Reported to the RNPMCHC for a check-up / Reported to another medical institution for a check-up / Received information from the information desk / Received information from relatives / Reported to the branch for inpatient treatment / Home visit / Examination by a district medical officer).

Field - Where the patient reported to (selectable by the list of medical institutions classifier).

Field - Control date (dd.mm.yyyyy)

Field - Form of control (Examination at the oncology branch / Observation at the medical institution at the place of residence / Examination at the medical institution by a mobile team / Examination at the RSNPMCHC / Examination at another medical institution / Inpatient treatment at the oncology branch).

Editing a patient record

You can edit or delete any card in the PCP system. You can also add additional data on treatment, checkup, second tumor, etc. to the card. At the same time, editing of the card is limited, depending on the user's access rights.

Drafts

The system should treat the patient's chart as a draft if there are certain errors (gross and soft):

-There are no clinical groups

-Discovery conditions 0-4

-Blank date of diagnosis.

All drafts of the system are contained in a separate section and are not taken into account in statistical calculations. They are visible in searches and lists. After correcting errors and saving the changes made, the patient record is transferred to the general system.

§4.4 Generating lists

The Lists section allows you to store sets of oncology patient charts organized by some feature and quickly navigate between them.

This section consists of three subsections:

-My Lists - lists created by the user.

-Available lists - lists created by other system users, which are marked as "Public list" and are available for viewing.

-All Lists - all lists to which the user has access.

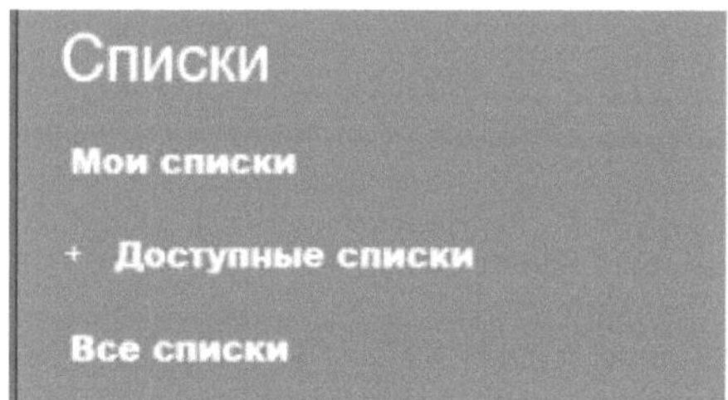

List view modes

List view modes allow you to switch the list to one mode or another:

-Patients - implies a list of all patients without cases

-Cases - allows to see all cases for each oncologic patient, i.e. if a card contains several records that meet the conditions of list formation, the system will display information on this card twice.

-Duplicates - the system will only display patients that contain 2 or more cases (primary-multiple), with one patient displayed on a single line.

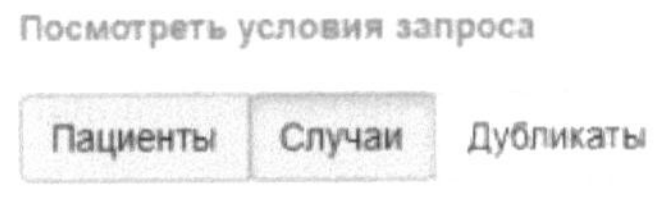

List conditions

When a list is created based on a search result, the following conditions can be viewed when the list is saved:

-List Name ;

List table name (for Researcher, Administrator, and Super Administrator);

-SQL query by which it was generated (for Super Administrator);

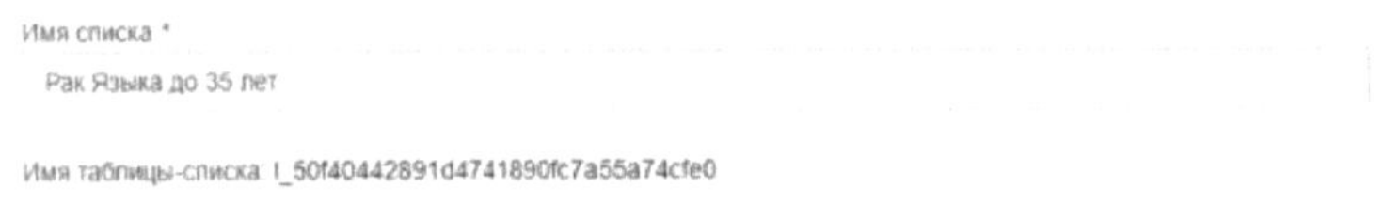

List handling

The PKR system implements several basic functions for working with lists:

- ***Creating lists***

Creating a simple list

Search based on a list (already created)

Copying search terms

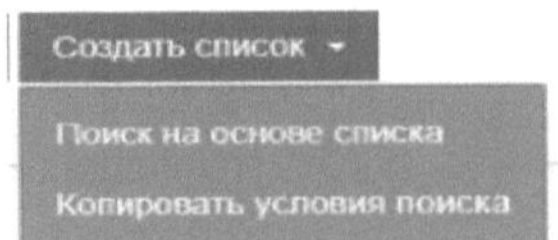

➢ ***Searching, editing and copying a list***

The list search function allows you to find a list with a specific title by the words specified in the search query. The search is performed for all sections: My Lists, Available Lists, All Lists.

The edit and copy functions are available for the Available Lists section, while the delete function is only available for the My Lists section.

➢ ***Operations with list data - Actions***

- Merge (2 or more lists) - used to merge lists when comparing created lists with the same conditions in different periods/years

-Subtract (2 or more lists) - used when retrieving lists with a "narrow" condition that cannot be retrieved in a simple query.

-Intersection (2 or more lists) - used to get a list with a certain condition from several lists.

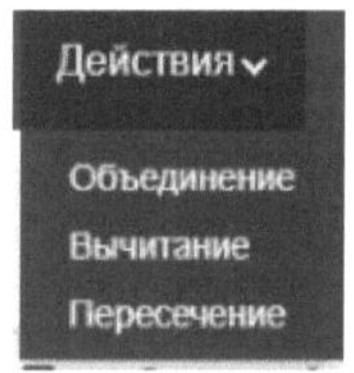

➢ ***Output of card/list information***

The Output function allows you to get information on card(s), lists presented in a certain way. This information can be viewed and printed as well as saved in Word format.

Note: This feature is active in the lists section, on a specific list page, and on a specific patient's card page.

Depending on which section of the system the user is in, the system will display a list of available output forms:

-Branch Call - Calling patients to a branch of the RSNPMCRC for examination or treatment.

-Extract - Extract 027-1/y-12 from the medical record of an inpatient (outpatient) patient with malignant neoplasm.

-Request to district oncologist - request to district oncologist about the fate of patients.

-Notification - notification of a first-time diagnosed case of malignant neoplasm.

-Brief Form - customizable form to display information such as name, date of birth, outpatient record #, address, diagnoses, patient fate.

-Protocol of neglect - protocol for when a patient is diagnosed with a neglected form of malignant neoplasm.

-Advanced form - basic patient information in a condensed form, including diagnosis and treatment.

- ***Import to the PKR database***

The Import function allows you to create new lists in the database from external sources.

These functions are available to the Administrator and Super Administrator.

Import to database

The Import to DB function allows importing a list into the system based on an existing table in the database (e.g. annual download of the population received by the State Statistical Committee of Uzbekistan).

Import from file

The Import from file function allows importing the list into the system on the basis of files, in which IDN (Unique Identification Number of the PCR system) / full name and date of birth, ICD-10 Code have been previously entered, in order to continue working with the lists received from outside (for example, the list of patients undergoing a certain clinical protocol in order to clarify their fate).

§4.5 Creating statistical reports

The "Statistics" section allows you to create different types of reports by templates, includes three sections - State Statistical Reporting, Additional Reporting, Numbers and Mortality.

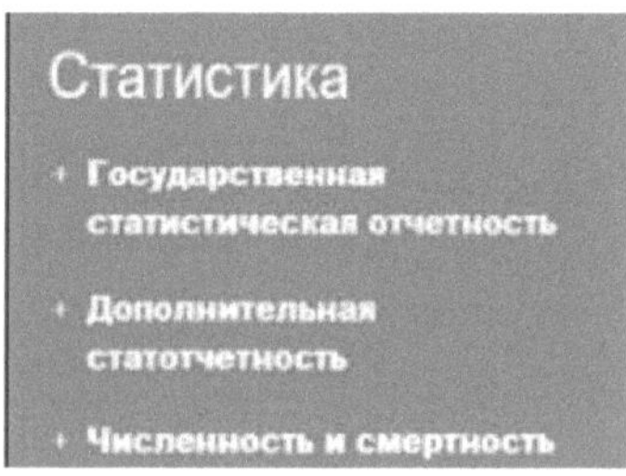

State statistical reporting

In this subsection the following forms of statistical reporting, which are part of the official state statistical form No. 7 "Information on diseases with malignant neoplasms", are distinguished:

Form 1-Children - Report on Medical Care for Children Section VII diseases in children aged 0-17 years.

Form 1-disease incidence - Report on the number of diseases registered in patients aged 18 years and older living in the service area of the health care organization providing therapeutic and preventive care.

Форма 1 заболеваемость

Дата формирования:

Отчет о числе заболеваний, зарегистрированных у больных в возрасте 18 лет и старше, проживающих в зоне обслуживания организации здравоохранения, оказывающей лечебно-профилактическую помощь

За 2021 год

Основные локализации	Число случаев заболеваний, зарегистрированных у лиц в возрасте 18 лет и старше		Из них с диагнозом, установленным впервые в жизни		Число лиц в возрасте 18 лет и старше, состоящих на диспансерном учете на конец отчетного периода	
	всего	из них у лиц старше трудоспособного возраста	всего	из них у лиц старше трудоспособного возраста	всего	из них у лиц старше трудоспособного возраста
Злокачественные новообразования – всего C00-C96						
из общего числа – злокачественные новообразования: губы C00						
пищевода C15						
желудка C16						
ободочной кишки C18						
прямой кишки C19-C21						
гортани C32						
трахеи, бронхов, легкого C33-C34						
костей и суставных хрящей C40-C41						
кожи C44						
молочной железы C50						
шейки матки C53						
тела матки C54						
яичника C56						
предстательной железы C61						
почки C64						
мочевого пузыря C67						
щитовидной железы C73						
болезнь Ходжкина C81						
неходжкинские лимфомы C82-C85						
множественная C88-C90						
лейкозы C91-C95						
Раки in situ – всего D00-D09						
из них шейки матки D06						
ВСЕГО C00-D09						

Form 2200 - Information on patients who died of MNs

Дата формирования:
Форма 2200
СВЕДЕНИЯ О ПАЦИЕНТАХ, УМЕРШИХ ОТ ЗЛОКАЧЕСТВЕННЫХ НОВООБРАЗОВАНИЙ
[Локализации (формы) злокачественных заболеваний]

Локализации (формы) злокачественных заболеваний			Число умерших в отчетном периоде	Из них дети в возрасте 0 - 17 лет	Из числа больных, у которых диагноз установлен в предыдущем году, умерло в течение одного года с момента установления диагноза
Злокачественные новообразования, всего	C00-C96	1	0	0	0
из них: губы	C00	2	0	0	0
полости рта	C01-C08	3	0	0	0
глотки	C09-C14	4	0	0	0
пищевода	C15	5	0	0	0
желудка	C16	6	0	0	0
ободочной кишки	C18	7	0	0	0
ректосигмоидного соединения, прямой кишки, ануса	C19-C21	8	0	0	0
печени и внутрипеченочных желчных протоков	C22	9	0	0	0
поджелудочной железы	C25	10	0	0	0
гортани	C32	11	0	0	0
трахеи, бронхов, легкого	C33,C34	12	0	0	0
костей и суставных хрящей	C40,C41	13	0	0	0
меланома кожи	C43	14	0	0	0
другие новообразования кожи	C44	15	0	0	0
соединительной и мягких тканей	C49	16	0	0	0
молочной железы	C50	17	0	0	0
шейки матки	C53	18	0	0	0
тела матки	C54	19	0	0	0
яичника	C56	20	0	0	0
предстательной железы	C61	21	0	0	0
почки	C64	22	0	0	0
мочевого пузыря	C67	23	0	0	0
центральной нервной системы	C70-C72	24	0	0	0
щитовидной железы	C73	25	0	0	0
болезнь Ходжкина (лимфогранулематоз)	C81	26	0	0	0
неходжкинские лимфомы	C82-C85	27	0	0	0
множественная миелома и иммунопролиферативные болезни	C88,C90	28	0	0	0
лейкозы	C91-C95	29	0	0	0
других локализаций (форм)		30	0	0	0

Form 2300 - Information on treatment of patients diagnosed with MN who are subject to special treatment.

Форма 2300

Дата формирования:

СВЕДЕНИЯ О ЛЕЧЕНИИ ПАЦИЕНТОВ С ДИАГНОЗОМ ЗЛОКАЧЕСТВЕННОГО НОВООБРАЗОВАНИЯ, ПОДЛЕЖАЩИХ СПЕЦИАЛЬНОМУ ЛЕЧЕНИЮ

За 2021 год

Локализации (формы) злокачественных заболеваний	Число больных, у которых диагноз установлен в отчетном периоде, закончивших специальное лечение по радикальной программе	Число больных, закончивших в отчетном периоде специальное лечение по радикальной программе	В том числе с использованием метода		
			только хирургического	только лучевого	только лекарственного
Злокачественные новообразования всего C00-C96 01	0	0	0	0	0
в том числе: губы C00 02	0	0	0	0	0
полости рта C01-C08 03	0	0	0	0	0
глотки C09-C14 04	0	0	0	0	0
пищевода C15 05	0	0	0	0	0
желудка C16 06	0	0	0	0	0
ободочной кишки C18 07	0	0	0	0	0
ректосигмоидного соединения, прямой кишки, ануса C19-C21 08	0	0	0	0	0
печени и внутрипеченочных желчных протоков C22 09	0	0	0	0	0
поджелудочной железы C25 10	0	0	0	0	0
гортани C32 11	0	0	0	0	0
трахеи, бронхов, легкого C33,C34 12	0	0	0	0	0
костей и суставных хрящей C40,C41 13	0	0	0	0	0
меланома кожи C43 14	0	0	0	0	0
другие новообразования кожи C44 15	0	0	0	0	0
соединительной и мягких тканей C49 16	0	0	0	0	0
молочной железы C50 17	0	0	0	0	0
шейки матки C53 18	0	0	0	0	0
тела матки C54 19	0	0	0	0	0
яичника C56 20	0	0	0	0	0
предстательной железы C61 21	0	0	0	0	0
почки C64 22	0	0	0	0	0
мочевого пузыря C67 23	0	0	0	0	0
центральной нервной системы C70-C72 24	0	0	0	0	0
щитовидной железы C73 25	0	0	0	0	0
болезнь Ходжкина (лимфогранулематоз) C81 26	0	0	0	0	0
неходжкинские лимфомы C82-C85 27	0	0	0	0	0
множественная миелома и иммунопролиферативные болезни C88,C90 28	0	0	0	0	0
лейкозы C91-C95 29	0	0	0	0	0

Form 7 - Distribution of cases of established MN by localization, sex and age.

Form 7a - Distribution of cases of first-time diagnosed malignant neoplasm by localization and patient age.

Additional statistical reporting

More than 90 statistical forms are included in this subsection, including crude, standardized, age-specific morbidity and mortality rates, crude and standardized errors, stage distribution, 1-year mortality rate, survival rates and their errors, treatment activity rates, and so on.

Population and mortality

This subsection includes several official forms on population size and mortality from the State Statistics Committee of the Republic of Uzbekistan.

Form 0301 - Distribution of population by sex and place of residence

Form 0302 - Distribution of population by age

Form 0304 - Distribution of mortality by sex and place of residence

Form 0305 - Distribution of population mortality by age

Working with reports

Work with reports includes: creating/deleting a report, viewing a report page, copying report keys, editing a report, Exporting to Word and Excel, as well as generating a list of patients according to a specified column of a statistical form.

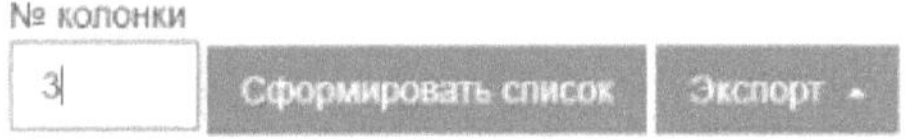

§4.6 Administration

The "Administration" section is intended for managing the PKP system, i.e. user accounts and roles. In addition, the section allows you to perform data audit and recovery procedures, IADI export, database comparison, database deletion, and error reporting.

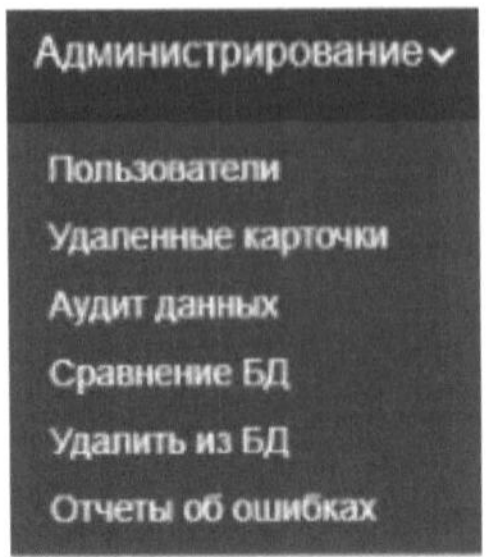

Active users

View the list of active/inactive users of the system. Responsible user - a user who is authorized to submit reports to the Ministry of Health (heads of organizational and methodological departments);

Ответственный	Состояние	Действия
+	Активен	
	Активен	
	Неактивен	
	Активен	
	Активен	
	Активен	
+	Активен	
+	Активен	
+	Активен	

Create informational notifications to the system users when work with the Database is performed, specifying the time from which the application will be unavailable to users (Super Administrator);

The super administrator manages the accounts of all users on the system:

Creates a user profile

Edits the profile

Changes the user password (if the user has forgotten his Login and password and was automatically locked out by the system)

Deletes user lists and reports

Users and their roles in the system

For distribution of access levels in the system different user roles are provided depending on the functionality available to them (Table 4.1).

The main roles of the system are:

-Researcher

-Student

-Registrar

-Administrator

-Superadministrator

Table 4.1.

Roles and rights of users of the Population Chancery Registry

Users	Rights and roles
Researcher, Intern, RMI/GMO Registrar, Regional Branch Office Registrar, RMI/GMO Administrator, Regional Branch Office Administrator, RMI/GMO Superadministrator, Regional Branch Office Superadministrator	Viewing patient records of any OB; Search for patient records of any regional branch; Simple search; Information Retrieval; Lists: -Creating , editing, deleting your lists -View available lists Reports: -Creating , editing, deleting your reports -View, export available reports -Output Forms: -View, export output form by patient, list
Researcher, Intern, Registrar in RMO/GMO, Registrar in Regional Branch Office	Regulated search, except for the section "Additional listings for analyzing information"

Administrator in RMI/GMO, Administrator in Regional Branch, Super Administrator in RMI/GMO, Super Administrator in Regional Branch	Regimented searches, including a section on "Additional Lists for Analyzing Information"; Data Audit; Database Comparison Deletion from the database
Registrar at the RMO/GMO, Registrar at the regional branch, Administrator in RMI/GMO, Administrator in Regional Branch, Super Administrator in RMI/GMO, Super Administrator in Regional Branch	Editing fragments such as "Dispensary notes", "Information about neglect", "Information about referral to other HMOs" in the patient card of the region of your RMO/GMO or regional branch; Saving a map as a Draft and being able to view drafts
Registrar in RMI/GMO, Administrator in RMI/GMO, Super Administrator in RMI/GMO	Limited editing of the passport part in the patient record of the patient's region of his/her RMO/GMO or regional affiliate
Registrar in the regional branch Administrator in the regional branch Superadministrator in a regional branch office	Complete map editing in your regional branch and area -Transferring patient records to your regional branch and region -Create a patient card in your regional branch and region -Deletion of patient records in your regional branch and area
Administrator in RMO/GMO, Administrator in Regional Branch Office	Working with the user: -View, create, edit user in their RMO/GMO, regional branch and region (except super admin); Lists: View IDN list
Superadministrator in RMO/GMO, Superadministrator in regional branch office	Working with the user: -View, create, edit user, including superadministrator, in their RMO/GMO, regional branch and region Lists: View SQL query

Data audit

The Data Audit feature will allow you to view information about user activity on the system and changes made to the system, such as:

-Addendum

-Editing

-Removal

Database Comparison

The Database Comparison function will allow you to compare existing databases with external databases to identify discrepancies (undercounted cases, diagnosis changes, etc.).

Note: This feature is available to Republican-level Administrator and Superadministrator.

Delete from database

The Delete from DB function will allow you to delete a large number of records from the database at the same time.

Error reports

The Error Reports function will allow you to create reports on the total number of errors that were made when creating or storing maps according to specified parameters.

IADI exports

The function of exporting information from the PKR system will allow to upload data according to a specific format for IARC.

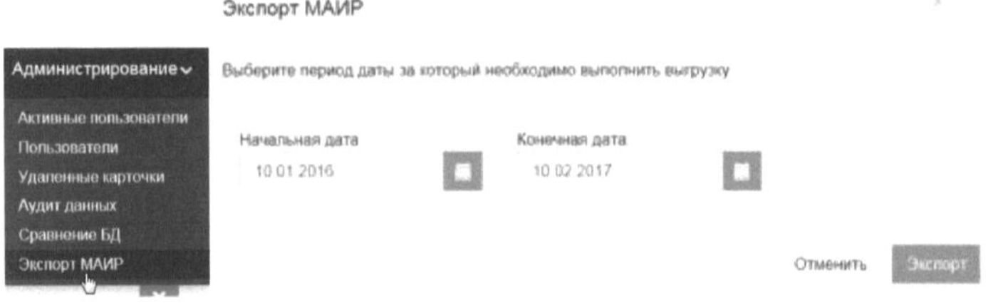

Note: This feature is available to the Republican SuperAdministrator.

- **<u>Example file for exporting to IARC:</u>**

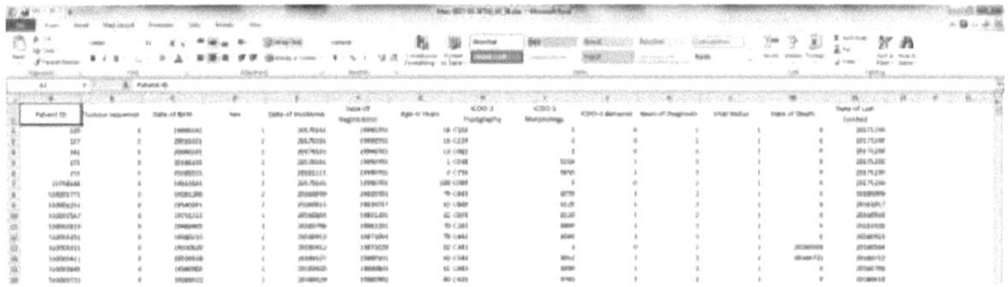

<u>Cell Value:</u>

✓ **Patient ID** - patient identification number in the system (corresponds to the IDN field);

✓ **Tumor sequence** - tumor (Numb_tum);

✓ **Date** of Birth - date of birth in the format YYYYYYYMMDD (corresponds to the Date Birth field);

✓ **Sex** - patient's gender; value 1 is male, value 2 is female;

✓ **Date of Incidence** - date of **incidence** in the format YYYYYYMMDD (corresponds to the Date Incid field);

✓ **Date of** Registration - date of registration in the format YYYYYYYMMDD (corresponds to the Date Regist field);

✓ **Age in Years** - patient's age (corresponds to the Agediag field);

✓ **ICDO-3 Topography** - code of diagnosis, according to the International Classification of Diseases (corresponds to the field ICD10);

✓ **ICDO-3 Morphology** - morphology code (corresponds to the MORPHOLOGY field);

✓ **ICDO-3 Behavior** - morphological behavior code (corresponds to the BHV field);

✓ **Basis of** Diagnosis - method of diagnosis confirmation (corresponds to the Bas Diag field);

✓ **Vital Status** - value of the patient's vital status (corresponds to the Vit Stat field - contains the following values: 1 - alive, 2 - dead);

✓ **Date of Death** - patient's date of death in YYYYYYMMDD format (corresponds to the Date Death field);

✓ **Date of Last Contact** - the date of the patient's last visit in the format YYYYYYMMDD (corresponds to the Date Visit field).

Integration of the stationery register with other databases

When creating a new patient chart, the system will integrate and search for the relevant information in the linked database. With this option, the system will automatically copy all patient information (Passport Part, General Diagnosis Information, IGC, etc.) from the linked database. Depending on the section, the copied information can be edited before or after it is saved.

Summary

The developed structure and methodology of the PCR are the basis for the functioning of the system, which includes: recording and maintaining information about the patient (primary and registered in the oncological institution); searching outpatient records of patients according to various parameters; forming and working with lists; obtaining various statistical reports and ensuring the availability of retrospective and current information from the PCR.

CHAPTER V. STATISTICAL INDICATORS USED IN THE POPULATION CANZER REGISTRY

There are specific statistical indicators that are used in population-based cancer registry. It is worth noting that in general medical statistics there is no section of statistical indicators used in oncology service. On this basis, a number of statistical indicators have been identified to assess the effectiveness of the organization of the oncological service, as well as anti-cancer measures, with a detailed description of the scope of their application [4, 6, 12, 18, 19, 20, 23, 24, 27, 31, 39, 41, 41, 44, 57, 58, 58, 63, 66, 65, 67, 67, 68, 71, 74, 75, 76, 77, 83, 84, 88, 99].

Table 5.1 categorized the statistical indicators of the cancer service into 7 main blocks:

- Indicators of primary morbidity of MN
- Mortality rates from MN
- Indicators of the organization of dispensary registration
- Indicators of the organization of treatment work
- Indicators of the status of timely diagnosis
- Quality indicators of population preventive examinations and screening programs
- Indicators for assessing the long-term results of treatment

Table 5.1.

Statistical indicators used in the oncology service

Indicators	Scope of the indicator
Indicators of primary morbidity of MN	
Number of first-time MN cases	Monitoring the increase in the number of MN diseases. Planning the organization of cancer control

Structure (extensive indicators) of MN morbidity (%)	Determination of priority directions of organization of anti-cancer fight
Crude intensive MN incidence rates (per 100,000 population)	Monitoring the growth of morbidity. Planning the organization of anti-cancer fight
Age-standardized intensive MN incidence rates (per 100,000 population)	Monitoring the growth of morbidity for different age groups. Planning the organization of cancer control
Standardized MN incidence rates (per 100,000 population)	Monitoring the growth of morbidity due to risk factors. Planning the organization of cancer control
Mortality rates from MN	
Number of deaths from ST in the reporting period	Monitoring the number of MN deaths. Planning the organization of cancer control
Structure (extensive indicators) of mortality from ST (%)	Determination of priority directions of organization of anti-cancer fight
Crude intensive MN mortality rates (per 100,000 population)	Monitoring of mortality dynamics for planning the organization of cancer control organization
Age-standardized intensive MN mortality rates (per 100,000 population)	Monitoring of mortality dynamics for planning the organization of cancer control organization
Standardized mortality rates from MN (per 100,000 population)	Comparative analysis of the effectiveness of cancer control programs in the regions. Integral assessment of the quality of cancer control organization
Total mortality (%)	Integral assessment of the organization of diagnostic and treatment work
Ratio of MN mortality to MN morbidity based on crude intensive indicators	Comparative analysis of the effectiveness of cancer control programs in the regions. Integral assessment of the quality of cancer control organization

Ratio of MN mortality to MN morbidity based on standardized indicators	Comparative analysis of the effectiveness of cancer control programs in the regions. Integral assessment of the quality of cancer control organization
Indicators of the organization of dispensary registration	
Percentage of patients who have undergone dispensary examination (%)	Estimation of patients' dispensary coverage (control level not less than 90%)
Percentage of patients of clinical group III who underwent dispensary examination (%)	Estimation of the coverage of patients cured of MN by dispensary (control level not less than 90%)
Percentage of patients observed for 5 or more years who have undergone dispensary examination (%)	Estimation of the coverage of long-term registered patients by dispensary (control level not less than 90%)
Indicators of the organization of treatment work	
Percentage of radical treatment coverage of curable patients (%)	Evaluation of the organization of treatment work. (benchmark level of at least 90%).
Percentage of incidence of radical surgical treatment of curable patients (%)	General assessment of surgical activity of oncologic dispensaries with differentiation by tumor process stages and tumor localizations (control level is determined by the best indicator among oncologic institutions according to the results of the previous year)
Percentage of frequency of combined and complex treatment with surgical component of curable patients (%)	Assessment of the organization of medical care with differentiation by tumor process stages (the reference level is determined by the best indicator among oncological institutions according to the results of the previous year)

Frequency of patients refusing radical treatment (%)	Assessment of the quality of explanatory and psychological work with patients (the benchmark level is determined by the best indicator among oncologic institutions based on the results of the previous year)
Frequency of common contraindications to radical treatment (%)	Assessment of the level of intensive care and resuscitation and anesthesia care (benchmark level is determined by the best indicator among oncologic institutions according to the results of the previous year)
Indicators of the status of timely diagnosis	
Proportion of patients with stages I and II of MN disease among those diagnosed for the first time (%)	Assessment of the organization of diagnostic work (control level is determined by the best indicator among oncological institutions according to the results of the previous year)
Frequency of late diagnosis (%)	Assessment of the organization of oncological care for the population, (the reference level is determined by the best indicator among oncological institutions according to the results of the previous year)
One-year mortality (%)	Assessment of the organization of timely diagnosis of MN (benchmark level is determined by the best indicator among oncological institutions based on the results of the previous year)
Quality indicators of population preventive examinations and screening programs	
Frequency of early detection of MN during preventive examinations of the population (%)	Assessment of the quality of screening and preventive examinations of the population (the benchmark level is determined by the best indicator among oncological institutions

	according to the results of the previous year)
Effectiveness of preventive examinations of the population (%)	Assessment of the quality of screening and preventive examinations of the population (the benchmark level is determined by the best indicator among oncological institutions according to the results of the previous year)
Frequency of in situ cancer detection (%)	Evaluation of the organization of early diagnosis and quality of screening programs (the benchmark level is determined by the best indicator among oncological institutions based on the results of the previous year)
Efficiency of women's examination rooms (%)	Overall assessment of the organization of work of women's examination rooms (benchmark level is determined by the best indicator among oncological institutions based on the results of the previous year)
Ratio of pre-invasive to invasive cervical cancer among those diagnosed through preventive screening (coefficient)	Assessing the quality of preventive screening of women (Work is considered effective when the index > 1.3)
Frequency of refusal of preventive examination of persons who were subsequently diagnosed with malignant tumor in the advanced stage (abs. number and %)	Quality indicator of explanatory and psychological work with patients (control level is determined by the best indicator among oncologic institutions according to the results of the previous year)
Indicators for assessing the long-term results of treatment	
Overall survival rate (%)	Integral indicator of cancer control organization
Adjusted survival (%)	Integral indicator of cancer control organization; Private indicator for assessing the effectiveness of treatment

	options for different groups of patients (reference level is determined by the best indicator among oncologic institutions according to the results of the previous year)
Relative survival rate (%)	Comparative integral indicator of the quality of organization of anti-cancer fight in separate territories. Private indicator for assessing the effectiveness of treatment options for different groups of patients (reference level is determined by the best indicator among oncologic institutions according to the results of the previous year)
Relative standardized survival rate (%)	Comparative integral indicator of the quality of organization of anti-cancer fight in separate territories. Private indicator for assessing the effectiveness of treatment options for different groups of patients (reference level is determined by the best indicator among oncologic institutions according to the results of the previous year)

Summary

The system of statistical indicators for oncology has some peculiarities, although in general it corresponds to the principles of medical statistics. In this chapter, a set of special indicators is formed to characterize the state of diagnosis and treatment of malignant neoplasms. Calculation and use of the indicators presented in the chapter on the basis of the state statistical reporting data is not possible, which once again confirms the necessity to create a population-based stationer-register.

CONCLUSION

Currently, there is an increase in the incidence of malignant neoplasms (MN) all over the world, as well as in the Republic of Uzbekistan (RUzb). Thus, according to the data of the state statistical reporting in the Republic of Uzbekistan in 2021, 25,578 new cases of MN were detected. Over the last 5 years, the number of first-time detected cases has increased by 12.5%. The incidence of MN per 100,000 population in RUzb reached 74.0, which is 14.2% higher than 5 years ago. At the same time, breast, gastric and cervical diseases have taken the first places in the general structure of MN morbidity over the last few years.

According to the International Agency for Research on Cancer (IARC), malignant tumors are a common disease with a relatively high mortality rate worldwide. Projection data from IARC and the World Health Organization (WHO), available on the Cancer Today 2020 website, show significant differences in incidence rates by country. In countries in the European region, incidence rates range from 148.1 per 100,000 population (Albania) to 372.8 (Ireland) (standardized rates, Standard World). In Asian countries, rates range from 80.9 (Nepal) to 285.1 (Japan) per 100,000 population. The North American continent has higher incidence rates than the European region in both the United States (362.2) and Canada (348.0). According to IARC-WHO projections, Uzbekistan has an incidence rate of 108.1 per 100,000 population in 2020, which is higher than Tajikistan (89.7 per 100,000 population) but lower than Afghanistan (108.8), Pakistan (110.4), Turkmenistan (128.8), Kyrgyzstan (130.6) and Kazakhstan (166.9).

The average mortality rate (standardized rate) in the world is projected to be 100.7 per 100,000 population in 2020. The lowest mortality rate was projected for Saudi Arabia (51.3 per 100,000 population) and the highest for Moldova (176.2). At the same time, in all countries the ratio of mortality to morbidity (based on standardized indicators) is quite high, which indicates the seriousness of the problem of radical treatment of MN. In the Republic of Uzbekistan, as in most Asian countries, this indicator exceeds 60%.

Each country has its own system of medical care for patients with MN. In turn, a vertical system has been created in RUzb in order to provide rational specialized medical care to cancer patients. Family physicians refer patients with suspected oncology to district oncologists. Oncologists of RMOs/GMOs keep records and monitor the condition of cancer patients in the district and provide primary care when necessary. In case of suspected oncology, they refer patients to regional oncology branches of the RSNPMCHC, where in-depth examination and treatment are carried out. If necessary, using telemedicine, consiliums are held with the participation of qualified specialists from RNNPMCRC and/or patients are issued a warrant for treatment at RNNPMCRC.

Correct and comprehensive registration of all MN cases according to international requirements is possible only if a population-based cancer registry is established.

The capabilities, goals and objectives of hospital-based and population-based cancer registries need to be clearly distinguished. Hospital-based registries do not collect information on patients with MN tied to a specific area, but only register patients with MN diseases treated at a specific health care facility. Therefore, the purpose of hospital registries is to assess the performance, planning and management of a single health facility. Detailed information about patients in hospital registries, diagnostic and treatment outcomes are the basis for scientific analysis. However, hospital registries, as a rule, are not engaged in tracking the fate of patients and, due to the incompleteness of recording all cases of MN at the territorial level, are not able to provide information on MN morbidity, mortality from MN, dispensary and treatment results. For this purpose, population-based cancer registries are organized, which register all cases of MN diseases at the territorial level and make it possible to collect statistical data.

The main distinguishing feature of population-based cancer registries from statistical reporting is the availability of detailed information about each patient with MN. The availability of such information has two significant advantages: the possibility of adding and correcting data about patients in the process of their observation, which in turn improves the quality of the entered information; the possibility of long-term follow-up of patients' fate and the availability of survival data. Statistical reports, which are collected from primary medical records, have a sufficient number of deficiencies, due to the delay in obtaining information on registered cases and further refinement of it in the process of examination and treatment. The basic principle of oncologic statistics is to collect and correct data on patients with MN diseases within several years after registration. For this reason, almost all foreign articles publish not quite "fresh" statistical data.

Today, statistical information is the main part of various cancer control programs. Data on morbidity and mortality are important for assessing the effectiveness of MN prevention, early and timely diagnosis of MN, screening programs, as well as for evaluating the effectiveness of various targeted interventions, since the main criterion for their successful application at the population level is the change in the levels of morbidity, mortality, survival and a number of other index indicators.

The planning of cancer control measures in RUzb, as well as the analysis of cancer patient survival at the population level will become possible after the organization of a population cancer registry in the country according to international standards. In the framework of this study, work was carried out to develop a methodology for a population-based cancer registry in RUzb.

The development of the methodology of the population-based cancer registry was based on the IARC-WHO recommendations: sources of information on first-time cases of MN (accounting forms of the Ministry of Health of the Republic of Uzbekistan), coding and confirmation of cases (ICD-10 and ICD-O-3), diagnosis (laboratory and instrumental diagnostic methods available in the country), treatment methods (in accordance with national standards of treatment of MN patients), statistical indicators to assess the prevalence of MN and the quality of services provided to patients with MN.

The material for studying the oncological situation in the Republic of Uzbekistan was the data obtained from the state reporting form (7) - the absolute number of first detected cases of MN in 2020. To analyze the oncological situation for 2020 in Bukhara oblast, data from Form 7 and personalized information from the primary documentation of the Bukhara branch of the RSNPMCHC&R were used. Standardization of morbidity indicators was carried out by the direct method using the world population standard (World Standard).

In 2020, 21,976 (2019 - 24,648) cases of MN were diagnosed for the first time in RUzb, including 9,059 cases diagnosed among men and 12,917 among women. The crude intensive MN incidence rate was 64 per 100,000 population. The highest MN incidence rates for 2020 were for breast cancer (9.8 per 100,000 population), stomach cancer (5.1), and cervical cancer (4.8).

Bukhara oblast was selected to assess the quality of organization of oncological care in RUzb. Bukhara oblast consists of 11 rural districts and 2 cities. The population of Bukhara oblast at the end of 2020 amounted to 1,923,934, i.e. 5.7% of the total population of the republic.

In Bukhara oblast there are 15 oncologic offices in the districts of the oblast. Staff positions of district oncologists in Bukhara oblast are 20.5 rates, of which 17.25 are employed. Of the working oncologists in the district polyclinics of Bukhara oblast (19 doctors), 90% of them have specialization in oncology.

As a result of work with primary medical documentation, a personalized database of patients was created. Analysis of the database allowed to identify a number of deficiencies in filling out and maintaining primary documentation. In the record forms there is often a tendency to fill in primary-multiple oncologic diseases (code C97 in ICD-10), without specifying the exact topography of each MN. It should be noted that each case in primary-multiple MNs should be registered as a separate case. A frequent mistake was the presence of notifications when a patient was diagnosed with precancerous (obligate) disease (clinical group Ia and Ib). Notices and extracts from the medical records of inpatients are written illegibly, with abbreviations of the patient's initials, date of birth, diagnosis and treatment. Moreover, the full clinical diagnosis is not always written (there is no precise indication of MN localization), in case of MN of one of the paired organs the side of the lesion is often not indicated, in the presence of metastases the exact organ of the lesion is not indicated. When staging MN, the stage according to the domestic classification (I-IV) and clinical group are not specified. The correct determination of the stage plays an important role in the selection of treatment methods. Based on the analyzed material, we can see that in 11.7% of cases the treatment tactics could be selected incorrectly. An important role in determining further treatment is played by pTNM, which due to the lack of a population cancer registry it is not possible to analyze. Besides, the staging of the disease according to the generally accepted clinical classification (I-IV) in

Bukhara region is done without letter specification (Ia-c, IIa-c, etc.), which also plays an important role in the choice of appropriate treatment.

According to the data collected, 1,584 cases of MN were identified for the first time in Bukhara oblast in 2020: 715 (45.1%) among men and 869 (54.9%) among women. The crude intensive MN incidence rate in Bukhara oblast in 2020 was 82.3 per 100,000 population.

In the structure of oncologic diseases of the population of Bukhara oblast the leading positions were occupied by: breast (16.0%), colorectal (6.6%) and stomach (6.0%).

Analyzing cancer morbidity by age, it should be noted that a significant increase in this indicator begins with the age group of 45-49 years, the peak incidence is observed among MN patients aged 75-79 years (577.3 per 100,000 population).

Analyzing the structure of oncological morbidity among all first diagnosed MNs by age, it should be noted that in Bukhara oblast up to 30 years of age, hemoblastoses (31.6%), brain MNs (10.5%), bone and joint MNs (8.6%) prevailed. In the age group of 30-44 years - MN of breast (29,3%), lymphomas (9,8%) and brain (9,3%). In patients in the age group of 45-64 years, breast (19.9%), cervical (7.0%) and gastric (6.8%) MNs were frequently registered. At the same time, skin (11.9%), lung (10.1%), and breast (8.0%) MNs were more frequently registered among older patients.

Comparative analysis of standardized morbidity rates of MN in Bukhara region showed that the standardized morbidity rate calculated using the world standard (88.7±2.3 per 100,000 population) is slightly higher ($p>0.05$) than the crude intensive rate (82.3±4.1 per 100,000 population), while the morbidity rate calculated using the African standard (56.7±1.5 per 100,000 population) is significantly lower ($p<0.001$). Significant scatter of both standardized and crude intensive indicators, as well as rather large standard errors of indicators indicate some errors in the available system of MN registration in Bukhara oblast.

The main purpose of the PCR in RUzb is to keep personalized records with regular follow-up of a patient with MN, as well as to keep records of first diagnosed cases of MN, and to keep information on the treatment provided.

The objectives of the SCR also include:

8. Registration of MN cases and their further completion, i.e. information on treatment - correct adherence to standards and protocols of treatment, diagnostics - correct diagnosis and dispensary. Quality control of the entered data.

9. Researching and conducting analysis of available data followed by the preparation of various reports.

10. Generalization of information in the RPC for the formation of state statistics for subsequent submission to the Ministry of Health.

11. Formation of annual analytical statistical compilations of the oncology service.

12. Conducting scientific, epidemiological, and government research programs that are necessary to improve cancer care in the country.

13. Protect and maintain existing and retrospective data in the RPC.

14. Opportunities for international scientific research.

The basic part of the RUzb RCT is the offices of district oncologists of RMOs/GMOs. Personal data on MN cases are sent from the district oncologist's office to the regional branches of the RNNPMCHC&R.

In the regional branches of RSPMCoIR, the RCD of RUzb functions in the form of registry offices, on the basis of organizational and methodological departments.

At the republican level, the RUzb RPC, in its turn, represents a branch of the Cancer Prevention Center, which is a part of the Cancer Prevention Center. This department is engaged in monitoring the activity of regional cancer registries, formation and submission of reports to the Ministry of Health of RUzb, assessment of oncology service, planning of anti-cancer activities in the regions and in the republic as a whole, assessment of onco-epidemiologic situation in each region, planning of procurement of expensive drugs and medical equipment, regular training seminars for medical personnel on international requirements for registration and registration of oncologic diseases. Based on this, the structure of the RPC was developed.

There are 5 main sections in the PKR system:

Search - section for searching for a patient in the card index according to the specified parameters.

New Patient - section for creating a card for a new patient

Lists - section for viewing and creating patient lists and working with drafts.

Statistics - section for the construction of state statistical and arbitrary statistical reporting in accordance with international requirements.

Administration - section for managing the PKP system (user accounts, rights and roles).

3 international reference books (International Classification of Diseases 10th revision (ICD-10); International Classification of Oncologic Diseases 3rd revision (ICD-O-3); TNM classification (latest revision)); Classification of Clinical Stages and 11 codifiers (System of designation of administrative-territorial object; Directory of registered professions in the republic; Directory of medical institutions registered in the republic; List of nationalities; Patient's condition; Side of lesion;

Clinical group; Method; Method of treatment) have been developed for PCR.

The blocks of statistical indicators for assessing the state of diagnostics and treatment of malignant neoplasms were also formed.

Statistical indicators of oncological service were divided into 7 main blocks: indicators of primary morbidity of MN; indicators of mortality from MN; indicators of dispensary registration organization; indicators of treatment work organization; indicators of timely diagnostics status; indicators of quality of preventive examinations of the population and screening programs; indicators of evaluation of long-term treatment results. For each group of indicators the scope of their application was defined, which plays an important role in the evaluation of anti-cancer measures.

CONCLUSIONS.

1. The conducted comprehensive analysis of the organization of oncological care for MN patients in the country allowed to identify an important link in the oncological service - oncological offices - staffing with oncologists will improve the quality and reliability of primary registration of MN patients, as well as the level of oncological alertness of the population. Oncoepidemiological analysis of morbidity of the population of the Republic of Uzbekistan for the last 10 years of MN revealed an increase in first-time MN cases by 15.6%, and the most typical for the country localizations of MN: breast (9.8 per 100 000 population), stomach (5.1) and cervix (4.8). The highest risk of developing MN is characteristic of the population aged 70-74 years (505, 7 per 100,000 population).

2. On the basis of the created population database of primary MN patients in Bukhara oblast the morbidity of the population was analyzed. The incidence of MN in Bukhara oblast was 82.3 per 100,000 population. In the structure of oncologic morbidity the leading positions were occupied by MNs of the breast (16.0%), colorectal zone (6.6%) and stomach (6.0%), the peak incidence occurred in the age group of 75-79 years (577.3 per 100 000 population). The analysis of the database revealed typical errors in the primary documentation: in 96 (11.7%) cases the stage was incorrectly determined, the most discrepancies were observed in the staging of pancreatic MN (32.1%), colorectal cancer (18.3%) and liver MN (15.1%). The most frequent error (46.9%) in establishing the clinical stage of the disease was the use of the numerical value of T category (TNM classification) as an indicator of clinical stage, so in 54.2% stage III was established instead of II and IV (40.6% and 12.5%, respectively).

3. The methodology of the population-based cancer registry was defined, and a list of directories (4 international) and codifiers (11 local) was formed and created, which is an integral part of the cancer registry and is necessary to obtain high-quality and reliable information on primary patients.

4. Indicators of oncological statistics are grouped into 7 basic blocks: indicators of primary morbidity of MN, indicators of mortality from MN, indicators of the organization of dispensary registration, indicators of the organization of treatment work, indicators of the state of timely diagnostics, indicators of the quality of preventive examinations of the population and screening programs, indicators of evaluation of the long-term results of treatment, which helps to assess the state of oncological care, the quality of services provided to the population, as well as to develop various programs

PRACTICAL RECOMMENDATIONS

1. It is recommended to analyze the quality and reliability of registration of MN patients in accordance with international requirements in order to assess the state of the oncology service and plan anticancer measures.

2. The developed list of variables, codifiers and reference books are recommended to be used in the implementation of population-based cancer registry in the Republic of Uzbekistan, as well as in the routine practice of specialists of oncology service.

3. When conducting oncoepidemiological and scientific studies, as well as when analyzing the quality of oncological care of the population, it is recommended to use the following groups of statistical indicators with a breakdown by the main localizations of MN, sex, age, periods, etc..:

✓ estimation of primary morbidity: absolute number of first-time MN cases, extensive, gross intensive, age and standardized morbidity indicators;

✓ estimation of MN mortality: absolute number of MN deaths, extensive, crude intensive, age-standardized and standardized mortality rates, total mortality rates, ratios of MN mortality to morbidity (based on absolute numbers/coarse/standardized);

✓ assessment of the organization of dispensary registration of MN patients: the proportion of patients who underwent dispensary examination, the proportion of patients of clinical group III who underwent dispensary examination, the proportion of patients observed for 5 or more years who underwent dispensary examination;

✓ assessment of the organization of treatment work: the percentage of coverage of radical treatment of curable patients, frequency of application of radical surgical treatment of curable patients, frequency of application of combined and complex treatment with surgical component of curable patients, frequency of patients' refusal of radical treatment, frequency of general contraindications to radical treatment;

✓ assessment of the organization of diagnostic work for timely detection of MN: the proportion of patients with stages I and II of the disease among newly diagnosed patients, the frequency of late diagnosis, one-year mortality;

✓ assessment of the quality of preventive examinations of the population and screening programs being developed: frequency of early detection of MN during preventive examinations of the population, efficiency of preventive examinations of the population, frequency of detection of cancer in situ, efficiency of women's examination rooms, ratio of pre-invasive and invasive forms of cervical cancer among persons diagnosed as a result of preventive examinations, frequency of refusal of preventive examinations of persons who are subsequently diagnosed with malignant cancer.

✓ Assessment of the long-term results of treatment of cancer patients: 1, 3, 5-year survival rates (overall, adjusted, relative).

LIST OF REFERENCES

1. Averkin Yu.I., Antonenkova N.N., Vejalkin I. V., Zalutsky I.V. Formation and development of the system of compulsory registration of new cases of malignant neoplasms in Belarus as a basis for the organization of anti-cancer fight // Oncological Journal. - 2007. - №1. - C. 74-81.

2. Algorithms of diagnosis and treatment of malignant neoplasms: clinical protocol / edited by O. G. Sukonko. - Ministry of Health of the Republic of Belarus. - Minsk: Professional edition, 2019. - 616 c.

3. Antonenko N.N., Zalutsky I.V., Averkin Y.I., Vejalkin I.V. Malignant neoplasms in the Republic of Belarus and their medical and social consequences // Onkolog. zhurn. - 2006. - T. 6, № 4. - C. 36-44.

4. Bogomaz V.M., Gorokh E.L., Lishishishina O.M., Ross G., Novichkova O. M., Stepanenko A.V. Indicators of the quality of medical care and their role in health care management // Ukrainian Med. chasopis. - 2010. - № 1. - C. 7-13.

5. Valkov M.Y., Karpunov A.A., Coleman M.P., Allemani K., Pankratieva A.Y., Potekhina E.F., Valkova L.E., Grzhibovsky A.M. Population Cancer Registry as a resource for science and practical health care // Human Ecology. - 2017. - №5. - C. 54-62

6. Glantz, S. Medico-biological statistics: Practice, -M. 1998. - 459 c.

7. Glushanko V.S., Gruzievich A.P., Garanicheva S.L., Alyakhnovich N.S., Kolbasich L.P. Fundamentals of medical statistics: textbook. - Vitebsk: VSMU, 2012. - 155 c.

8. Grinhalch T. Fundamentals of evidence-based medicine / per.s angl.ed. by I.N. Denisov, K.I. Saitkulov, V.P. Leonov. - 4th edition, revision and supplement. - M. : GEOTAR-Media, 2018. -336 c.

9. Zhizhin K.S. Medical statistics: Textbook. - Rostov N/D: Phoenix, 2007. - 160 c.

10. Malignant neoplasms in Russia in 2020 (morbidity and mortality) / Edited by A.D. Kaprin, V.V. Starinsky, A.O. Shakhzadova. Starinsky, A.O. Shakhzadova. - Moscow: P.A. Herzen MNIOI - branch of FGBU "NMRC Radiology" of the Ministry of Health of Russia, - 2021. - 252 c.

11. Kisteneva O.A., Nesterenko A.V., Byldina A.I. Oncology in the history of medicine // International scientific review. - 2017. - №1 - C. 32.

12. Konsybaeva K. E. Indicators of the quality of medical care // Medicine. - 2013. - № 4. - C. 5-7.

13. Kolomiichenko M.E. Criteria of accessibility and quality of medical care: normative regulation // Bulletin of the Semashko National Research Institute of Public Health. 2020. №3. C. 46-51.

14. Krekoten E. N. Justification of indicators of the quality of medical care of the stage "prevention" // Vestnik. VSMU. - 2013. - T. 12, № 4. - C. 129 - 132.

15. Lang T. A., Cecik M. How to describe statistics in medicine: a handbook for authors, editors and reviewers / translated from English. ed. by V. P. Leonov. P. Leonov. - Moscow: Prakt. medina, 2011. - 477 c.

16. Maksimov, D.A., Shepel E.V., Aseev A.V. History of formation and development of oncomammology // Issues of reconstructive and plastic surgery. - 2020. - №2(73). - C.72-78.

17. R.K. Makhmudov, O.A. Galfinger. Geoinformation analysis of socio-demographic development of the countries of Central Asia // Inter Carto Inter GIS.-2016. - C. 42-49.

18. Merabishvili V. M. Survival rate of oncologic patients - St. Petersburg : Kosta Publishing Polygraphic Company, 2006. -440 c.

19. Merabishvili V. M. Oncologic statistics (traditional methods, new information technologies). Manual for doctors: in 2 parts. - SPb : Kosta Publishing Polygraphic Company, 2011. - Part 2. - 247 p.

20. Merabishvili V.M. Oncologic statistics (traditional methods, new information technologies): A guide for physicians. Edition of the second, supplemented. Part I., 2015. - 223 c.

21. Methodology for calculating indicators of the activity of health care institutions and public health: training and methodological manual. - Stavropol, 2006. - 39 c.

22. Moiseev P. I., Veyalkin I.V., Demidchik Y.E. Epidemiology of malignant neoplasms: principles and methods / Manual of Oncology : in 2 vol. ; under general ed. by O. G. Sukonko . - Minsk: Belarus. encykl. imen P. Brovki, 2015. - T. 1. - Ch. 2. - 51-81 c.

23. Moiseev P.I., Yakimovich G.V., Okeanov A.E., Zubets O.I., Kirpichenko T.N. Cancer in Europe: a look at the problem, a comparative analysis of some indicators // Onkolog. zhurn. - 2014. - T. 8, № 3. - C. 13-23.

24. Okeanov A. E., Moiseev P. I., Evmenenko A. A. A., Levin L. F. 25 years against cancer. Successes and problems of anti-cancer fight in Belarus for 1990-2014 years / edited by O. G. Sukonko. - N.N. Aleksandrov RNPC MPA. - Minsk: GU RNMB, 2016. - 415 c.

25. Okeanov, A.E., Moiseev P.I., Levin L.F. Statistics of oncologic diseases in the Republic of Belarus (2006-2015) / edited by O.G. Sukonko. - Minsk: RNPC MPA named after N.N. Aleksandrov, 2016. - 280 c.

26. Fundamentals of evidence-based medicine. Textbook for the system of postgraduate professional education of doctors / Edited by Academician of the Russian Academy of Medical Sciences, Professor R.G. Oganov. - Moscow: Silicea-Pograf, 2010. - 136 c.

27. Petrova G.V., Gretzova O.P., Starinsky V.V.. Characteristics and methods of calculation of statistical indicators used in oncology. - Moscow: P.A. Herzen MNIOI, 2005. -39 c.

28. Polyakov S.M., Levin L.F., Shebeko N.G., Kirchinko T.I. Automated system of information processing of the Belarusian Chancery Register: technological instruction for the formation of the database of the Belarusian Chancery Register. - Minsk, 2006. - 44 c.

29. Decree of the President of the Republic of Uzbekistan No. PP-2866 dated April 4, 2017 "On measures for further development of oncological care for the population of the Republic of Uzbekistan for 2017-2021". - Tashkent, 2017. - 7 c.

30. Decree of the President of the Republic of Uzbekistan #PP-5130 dated May 27, 2021 "On further improvement of the system of providing hematology and oncology services to the population. - Tashkent, 2021. - 24 c.

31. Savelyev V. N. N., Vinogradova T. V., Dunayev S. M. Indicators of the quality of medical care // Med. almanac. - 2011. - № 1. - C. 11-14.

32. Sachek M.M., Filonyuk V.A., Malakhova I.V., Dudina T.V., Yolkina A.I. Evaluation of the effectiveness of scientific developments focused on practical health care (literature review) // Vopr. organization and informatization of health care. - 2013. -№ 1. - C. 13-32.

33. Health Systems: Time for Change. Australia. European Observatory on Health Systems - Internet resource: http://apps.who.int/iris/bitstream/10665/108466/2/E74466sumR.pdf.

34. State of oncological care to the population of the Republic of Uzbekistan in 2020 / edited by M.N. Tillyashayhov, Sh.N. Ibragimov, S.M. Dzhanklich. - Tashkent: IPTD "Uzbekistan", 2021. - 176 c.

35. State of oncological care to the population of the Republic of Uzbekistan in 2021 / edited by M.N. Tillyashayhov, Sh.N. Ibragimov, S.M. Dzhanklich. - Tashkent: IPTD "Khalk", 2022. - 176 c.

36. State of oncological care for the Russian population in 2020 / Edited by A.D. Kaprin, V.V. Starinsky, A.O. Shakhzadova. Starinsky, A.O. Shakhzadova. - Moscow: P.A. Herzen MNIOI - branch of FGBU "NMRC Radiology" of the Ministry of Health of Russia, 2021. - 239 c.

37. Standards of diagnostics and treatment of malignant neoplasms / community of authors. - Tashkent: "Complex print", 2022, - 507 p.

38. Sukonko O. G., Moiseev P. I., Okeanov A. E. Specialized medical care for cancer patients in 2013 according to the materials of the final meeting of chief physicians and specialists of oncological institutions of the Republic of Belarus // Onkolog. zhurn. 2014. - T. 8, № 1. - C. 5-16.

39. Khabriev R.U., Vorobyev P.A., Yuriev A.S., Nikonov E.L., Avksentyeva M.V. Indicators of the quality of medical care (regional level) // Probl. standardization in public health. - 2005. - № 10. - C. 54-63.

40. Heifets N. E. Improvement of the system of quality management of medical care in the Republic of Belarus at the present stage // Medical and social ecology of personality: status and prospects: materials of the X international conference, Minsk, 6-7 April. 2012 г. - Minsk : Izd. center BSU, 2012. - C. 326-328.

41. Yuryev A.S., Aksentyeva M.V., Vorobyev P.A., Gorbunov S.N. Methodological approaches to the formation of relevant indicators of the quality of medical care // Probl. standardization in public health. - 2005. - № 8. - C. 9-15.

42. Armstrong B. K. The role of the cancer registry in cancer control // Cancer Causes Control. - 1992. - Vol. 3, iss. 6. - pp. 569-579.

43. Babenko AI, Takhauov RM. Age-specific and gender characteristics of patterns of development of malignant malformations in Tomskaya oblast // Probl Sotsialnoi Gig Zdravookhranenniiai Istor Med. - 2006. - Vol. 1. - pp. 46-50.

44. Balawardena J, Skandarajah T, Rathnayake W, Joseph N. Breast Cancer Survival in Sri Lanka // JCO Glob Oncol. - 2020. - Vol. 6. - pp. 589-599. doi: 10.1200/JGO.20.00003.

45. Barchuk A, Belyaev A, Gretsova O, Tursun-Zade R, Moshina N, Znaor A. History and current status of cancer registration in Russia // Cancer Epidemiol. - 2021. Vol. 73. - pp. 963. doi: 10.1016/j.canep.2021.101963.

46. Barchuk A, Tursun-Zade R, Belayev A, Moore M, Komarov Y, Moshina N, Anttila A, Nevalainen J, Auvinen A, Ryzhov A, Znaor A. Comparability and validity of cancer registry data in the northwest of Russia // Acta Oncol. - 2021. - Vol. 60, №10. - pp. 1264-1271. doi: 10.1080/0284186X.2021.1967443.

47. Bashar MA, Thakur JS, Budukh A. Evaluation of Data Quality of Four New Population Based Cancer Registries (PBCRs) in Chandigarh and Punjab, North India- A Quality Control Study // Asian Pac J Cancer Prev. - 2021. - Vol. 22, № 5. - pp. 1421-1433. doi: 10.31557/APJCP.2021.22.5.1421.

48. Behera P, Patro BK. Population Based Cancer Registry of India - the Challenges and Opportunities// Asian Pac J Cancer Prev. - 2018. - Vol. 19, № 10. - pp. 2885-2889. doi: 10.22034/APJCP.2018.19.10.2885.

49. Bhatia A, Victora CG, Beckfield J, Budukh A, Krieger N. "Registries are not only a tool for data collection, they are for action":

Cancer registration and gaps in data for health equity in six population-based registries in India // Int J Cancer. - 2021. Vol. 148, № 9. - pp. 2171-2183. doi: 10.1002/ijc.33391.

50. Bierich R. Die Krebsbekampfung in Hamburg. In: Gruneisen, F. /ed. Jahrbuch des Reichsausschusses fur Krebsbekamfung. - Leipzig. - 1991. - 47 p.

51. Bray F, Colombet M, Mery L, Piñeros M, Znaor A, Zanetti R, Ferlay J. Cancer Incidence in Five Continents (IARC). - 2021.- Vol. XI.-#166. - 1543 p. Available from: https://publications.iarc.fr/597.

52. Bray F, Ferlay J, Laversanne M, Brewster DH, Gombe Mbalawa C, Kohler B, Piñeros M, Steliarova-Foucher E, Swaminathan R, Antoni S, Soerjomataram I, Forman D. Cancer Incidence in Five Continents: Inclusion criteria, highlights from Volume X and the global status of cancer registration. Int J Cancer. 2015 Nov 1;137(9). - 2060 p. doi: 10.1002/ijc.29670. PMID: 26135522.

53. Bray F, Parkin DM. Evaluation of data quality in the cancer registry: principles and methods. Part I: comparability, validity and timeliness // Eur J Cancer. - 2009. - Vol. 45, № 5. - pp. 747-55. doi: 10.1016/j.ejca.2008.11.032.

54. Bray F, Znaor A, Cueva P, Korir A, Swaminathan R, Ullrich A, Wang SA, Parkin DM. Planning and Developing Population-Based Cancer Registration in Low- or Middle-Income Settings. - Lyon. - 2014. - 46 p. PMID: 33502836.

55. Bray F., Jemal A., Grey N. , Ferlay J., Forman D. Global cancer transitions according to the human development index (2008-2030): a population-based study // The Lancet oncology. - 2012. Vol. 13, № 8. - pp. 790-801.

56. Cancer control strategy for Poland 2015-2024 Internet resource: https://www.iccp-portal.org/system/files/plans/Cancer%20Plan%20Poland.pdf

57. Cancer in Europe / Edited by Jemal A., Vineis P., Bray F., Torre L., D. Forman // The Cancer Atlas. - 2nd ed. - 2014. - pp. 56-57.

58. Cancer Registration: Principles and Methods / Edited by O.M. Jensen, D.M. Parkin, R. MacLennan, C.S. MuirandR.G. Skeet // IARC Scientific Publications No 95. - Lyon: IARC, 1991. - pp. 296.

59. Carmen Martos, Emanuele Crocetti (Coordinator), Otto Visser, Brian Rous, Francesco Giusti and the Cancer Data Quality Checks Working Group, A proposal on cancer data quality checks: one common procedure for European cancer registries - version 1.1, EUR 29089 EN, Publications Office of the European Union, Luxembourg.- 2018. - 99 p. doi:10.2760/429053

60. Charlton M, Schlichting J, Chioreso C, Ward M, Vikas P. Challenges of Rural Cancer Care in the United States. // Oncology (Williston Park). - 2015. - Vol. 9. - pp. 633-640

61. Clemmesen, J. Statistical studies in the etiology of malignant neoplasm. // ActaPathol. Microbiol. Scand. - 1965. - 1. - Suppl.174

62. de Martel C, Georges D, Bray F, Ferlay J, Clifford GM. Global burden of cancer attributable to infections in 2018: a worldwide incidence analysis // Lancet Glob Health. - 2020. - Vol. 8, № 2. - pp. e180-e190.

63. Dickman P. W., Hakulinen T. Survival analysis . - Tallinn : Institute of Experimental and Clinical Medicine Tallinn, 2000. - 248 p.

64. Dickman P. W., Hakulinen T, Luostarinen T, Pukkala E, Sankila R, Söderman B, Teppo L. Survival of cancer patients in Finland 1955-1994 // Acta Oncol. - 1999. - Vol. 38. - pp. 1-10.

65. Dyba T, Randi G, Bray F, Martos C, Giusti F, Nicholson N, Gavin A, Flego M, Neamtiu L, Dimitrova N, Negrão Carvalho R, Ferlay J, Bettio M. The European cancer burden in 2020: Incidence and mortality estimates for 40 countries and 25 major cancers // Eur J Cancer. - 2021. - Vol. 157. - pp. 308-347. doi: 10.1016/j.ejca.2021.07.039.

66. Estève J, Benhamou E, Croasdale M, Raymond L. Relative survival and the estimation of the net survival: elements for further discussion // Statistics in Medicine. - 1990. - Vol. 9, iss. 5. - pp. 529-538.

67. Faivre J, Bossard N, Jooste V; GRELL EUROCARE-5 Working Group. Trends in net survival from colon cancer in six European Latin countries: results from the SUDCAN population-based study // Eur J Cancer Prev. - 2017. - Vol. 26. - pp. S40-S47. doi: 10.1097/CEJ.0000000000000293.

68. Ferlay J, Colombet M, Soerjomataram I, Dyba T, Randi G, Bettio M, Gavin A, Visser O, Bray F. Cancer incidence and mortality patterns in Europe: Estimates for 40 countries and 25 major cancers in 2018 // Eur J Cancer. - 2018. - Vol. 103. - pp. 356-387. doi: 10.1016/j.ejca.2018.07.005

69. Ferlay J, Ervik M, Lam F, Colombet M, Mery L, Piñeros M, Znaor A, Soerjomataram I, Bray F (2020). Global Cancer Observatory: Cancer Today. Lyon, France: International Agency for Research on Cancer. Internet resource: https://gco.iarc.fr/today, doi: 10.1002/ijc.33588. Epub ahead of print. PMID: 33818764

70. International Health Care System Profiles. Internet resource: http://international.commonwealthfund.org/countries/germany/

71. Jönsson L, Sandin R, Ekman M, Ramsberg J, Charbonneau C, Huang X, Jönsson B, Weinstein MC, Drummond M. Analyzing overall survival in randomized controlled trials with crossover and implications

for economic evaluation // Value Health. - 2014. - Vol. 17, № 6. - pp. 707-713. doi: 10.1016/j.jval.2014.06.006.

72. Keding, J. Annotation zur Krebsepidemiologie. Humburg. Arzteblatt. - 1973. - 27 p.

73. Kennaway E.L.. The data relating to cancer in the publications of the General Register Office // Br. J. Cancer. - 1950. - №4. - pp. 158-172.

74. Mariotto A, Capocaccia R, Verdecchia A, Micheli A, Feuer EJ, Pickle L, Clegg LX. Projecting SEER cancer survival rates to the US: an ecological repression approach // Cancer Causes Control. - 2020. - Vol. 13, № 2. - pp. 101-111.

75. Palmqvist C, Staf C, Mateoiu C, Johansson M, Albertsson P, Dahm-Kähler P. Increased disease-free and relative survival in advanced ovarian cancer after centralized primary treatment // Gynecol Oncol. - 2020. - Vol. 159, № 2. - pp. 409-417. doi: 10.1016/j.ygyno.2020.09.004.

76. Parkin D. M., Hakulinen T. Analysis of survival. Cancer registration: principles and methods / ed.: O. M. Jensen. M. Jensen. - Lyon, France, 1991. - 296 p.

77. Parkin D.M, Bray F. Evaluation of data quality in the cancer registry: principles and methods Part II. Completeness // Eur J Cancer. - 2009. - Vol. 45, № 5. - pp. 756-64. doi: 10.1016/j.ejca.2008.11.033.

78. Pathways to health system performance assessment. A manual to conducting health system performance assessment at national or sub-national level. - Copengagen : WHO regional office for Europe. - 2018. - 86 p.

79. Plsek, P. E. Quality improvement methods in clinical medicine // Pediatrics. - 1999. - Vol. 103, № 1. - pp. 203-214.

80. Precer A. S., Harding A. The economics of public and private roles in health care // The international bank for reconstruction and development. - The World Bank, 2016. - 25 p.

81. Ramseook-Munhurrun P., Lukea-Bhiwajee S. D., Naidoo P. Services quality in the public service // Int. J. Manag. Market. Res. - 2010. - Vol. 3, № 1. - pp. 37-50.

82. Rechel B, Richardson E, McKee M. Trends in health systems in the former Soviet countries [Internet]. Copenhagen (Denmark): European Observatory on Health Systems and Policies; 2014. PMID: 28972708.

83. Reeves GK, Beral V, Bull D, Quinn M. Estimating relative survival among people registered with cancer in England and Wales // Br J Cancer. - 1999. - Vol. 79, № 1. - pp. 18-22. doi: 10.1038/sj.bjc.6690005.

84. Rezaianzadeh A, Jalali M, Maghsoudi A, Mokhtari AM, Azgomi SH, Dehghani SL. The overall 5-year survival rate of breast cancer among Iranian women: A systematic review and meta-analysis of published studies. // Breast Dis. - 2017, iss. 37 (2). - pp. 63-68. doi: 10.3233/BD-160244. PMID: 28655117.

85. Rozhavskiĭ LA. The medical demographic issues of the Leningradskaya Oblast // Probl Sotsialnoi Gig Zdravookhranenniiai Istor Med. - 2008 Jan-Feb. - pp. 5-8. PMID: 18649686.

86. Ryzhov A, Corbex M, Piñeros M, Barchuk A, Andreasyan D, Djanklich S, Ghervas V, Gretsova O, Kaidarova D, Kazanjan K, Mardanli F, Michailovich Y, Ten E, Yaumenenka A, Bray F, Znaor A. Comparison of breast cancer and cervical cancer stage distributions in ten newly independent states of the former Soviet Union: a population-based study // Lancet Oncol. - 2021, Vol. 22. - pp. 361-369. doi: 10.1016/S1470-2045(20)30674-4. Epub 2021 Feb 5. PMID: 33556324; PMCID: PMC8014987.

87. Sabesan, S. Brennan, S. . Tele Oncology for Cancer Care in Rural Australia. In: Graschew, G. , Rakowsky, S. , editors. Telemedicine Techniques and Applications // London: IntechOpen. - 2011. - pp. 289-306. Available from: https://www.intechopen.com/chapters/16886 doi: 10.5772/17112.

88. Sandin F. Analyzing and modeling the relative survival rate of patients diagnosed with malignant melanoma. Department of Mathematics Uppsala University. - 2008. - 39 p.

89. Schinz H.R.. Kleine Internationale Krebskonferenzvom 2-6 Sept. 1946 in Kopenhagen. Schweiz. Med. Wochenschr. 2016. - 76 p.

90. Shaw C. The external assessment of health services // World Hosp. Health Serv. - 2004. - Vol. 40, № 1. - pp. 24-27.

91. Sieveking G.H.. Das Krebs problem in deroffentlichen Gesundhietsfursorge. // Z. Gesamtwerwalt. Gesamtfursorge. - 2017. - №1. - pp. 23-30.

92. Sieveking G.H.. Die Hamburger Krebskranken fur rsorgeim Vergleichmitgleichyartigen in- und auslandischen Einrichtungen // Bull. Schweiz. Ver. Krebsbekampf. - 2018. - Vol.2. - pp. 115-123.

93. Sieveking G.H.. Die Hamburger Krebskrankenfurrsorge 1927-1932 // Z. Gesamtwerwalt. Gesamtfursorge. - 2019. - №4. - pp 241-247.

94. Sieveking G.H.. Hamburgs Krebskranken furrsorge 1927-1939 // Mschr. Krebsbekampf. - 2020. - №4. - pp. 49-52.

95. Sigurdardottir LG, Jonasson JG, Stefansdottir S, Jonsdottir A, Olafsdottir GH, Olafsdottir EJ, Tryggvadottir L. Data quality at the Icelandic Cancer Registry: comparability, validity, timeliness and completeness. // Acta Oncol. - 2012 Sep, - Vol 51(7). - pp. 880-900. doi: 10.3109/0284186X.2012.698751. PMID: 22974093.

96. Silva S. Cancer Epidemiology: Principles and Methods. - IARC, Lyon, France . - 1999. - 442 p.

97. Stocks P. Cancer registration and studies of incidence by surveys. // Bull. World Health Org. - 1959. - №20. - pp. 697-715.

98. Storm HH, Michelsen EV, Clemmensen IH, Pihl J. The Danish Cancer Registry--history, content, quality and use. Dan Med Bull. - 1997 Nov. - Vol.44(5).- 535 p. PMID: 9408738.

99. Tang H, Jiang X, Lou J, Chen T. Methodology for survival assessment of cancer patients using population-based cancer registration data // Zhejiang Da Xue Xue Bao Yi Xue Ban. - 2018 Jan 25.- 47(1).- pp. 104-109. Chinese. doi: 10.3785/j.issn.1008-9292.2018.02.15. PMID: 30146819.

100. The Canadian Strategy for Cancer Control: A Cancer Plan for Canada - online resource: https://www.partnershipagainstcancer.ca/wp-content/uploads/2017/09/canadian-strategy-for-cancer-control-a-cancer-plan-for-canada.pdf

101. Thoburn KK, German RR, Lewis M, Nichols PJ, Ahmed F, Jackson-Thompson J. Case completeness and data accuracy in the Centers for Disease Control and Prevention's National Program of Cancer Registries. // Cancer. - 2007 Apr 15.- iss 109(8).- pp.1607-1616. doi: 10.1002/cncr.22566. PMID: 17343277.

102. Torre LA, Siegel RL, Ward EM, Jemal A. Global Cancer Incidence and Mortality Rates and Trends--An Update // Cancer Epidemiol Biomarkers Prev. - 2016 Jan.- Vol.25.- No.1.- pp.16-27. doi: 10.1158/1055-9965.EPI-15-0578. Epub 2015 Dec 14. PMID: 26667886.

103. Vaktskjold A, Lebedintseva JA, Korotov DS, Tkatsjov AV, Podjakova TS, Lund E. Cancer incidence in Arkhangelskaja Oblast in northwestern Russia. The Arkhangelsk Cancer Registry. BMC Cancer. -

2005 Jul 19.- Vol.5.- 82 p. doi: 10.1186/1471-2407-5-82. PMID: 16029510; PMCID: PMC1181809.

104. Wagner, G. Cancer registration: Historical aspects. In: Parkin, D.M., Wagner, G. and Muir. C.S. eds., The Role of the Cancer Control. -IARC Scientific Publications. - 1985 (66) .- 12 p.

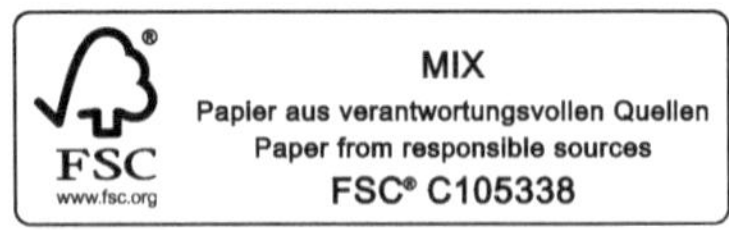

Printed by Books on Demand GmbH, Norderstedt / Germany